SECRETS OF
COLOUR
HEALING

STEPHANIE NORRIS

IVY PRESS

This edition published in the UK and North America in 2018 by
Ivy Press
An imprint of The Quarto Group
The Old Brewery, 6 Blundell Street
London N7 9BH, United Kingdom
T (0)20 7700 6700 **F** (0)20 7700 8066
www.QuartoKnows.com

First published in the UK in 2001

© 2017 Quarto Publishing plc

British Library Cataloguing-in-Publication Data
A catalogue record for this book is available from
the British Library

ISBN: 978-1-78240-537-5

This book was conceived, designed and produced by
Ivy Press
58 West Street, Brighton BN1 2RA, UK

Art Director: Peter Bridgewater
Publisher: Sophie Collins
Editorial Director: Steve Luck
Designers: Kevin Knight, Jane Lanaway and Ginny Zeal
Project Editor: Caroline Earle
Picture Researcher: Vanessa Fletcher and Trudi Valter
Photography: Guy Ryecart
Illustrations: Sarah Young and Michael Courtney
Three-dimensional Models: Mark Jamieson
Assistant Editor: Jenny Campbell

Printed in China

10 9 8 7 6 5 4 3 2 1

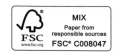

Cover image: Shutterstock/a_Jarm

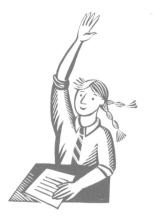

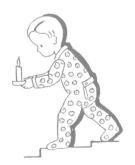
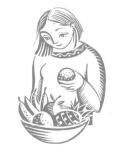
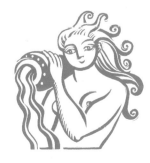

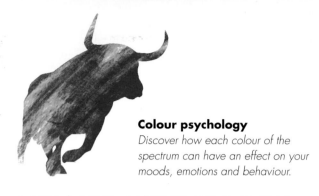

Colour psychology
*Discover how each colour of the
spectrum can have an effect on your
moods, emotions and behaviour.*

HOW TO USE THIS BOOK
To make this book easy to use it has
been split into four distinct sections. The first of these describes how colour was used
for healing in ancient times and explains the scientific principles behind colour healing.
The second part focuses on the seven colours of the spectrum and their properties. The
third part details the methods of colour healing, giving advice on practising colour
healing at home, including colour visualization and colour meditation. The final part
looks at how colour in the environment is important and how to feel in harmony
with the colours we absorb in our daily lives.

Further Information
Neither publisher nor author
can be held responsible for
any event, claim or belief
described in this book. If you
have a medical or psychiatric
condition, you are advised
to consult your doctor before
embarking on any course
of colour therapy. Colour
therapy is not intended to
be a substitute for any
medical, hospital or
psychiatric treatment.

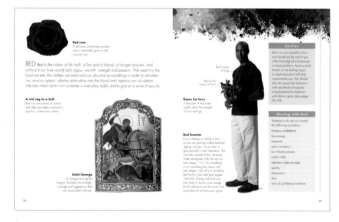

Practical information
*The properties of each colour are
described on colourful practical pages.*

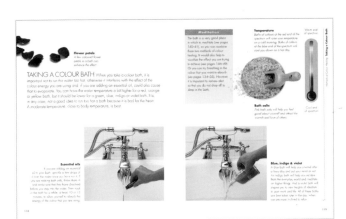

Home treatment
Practical spreads show how you can use various colour treatments at home.

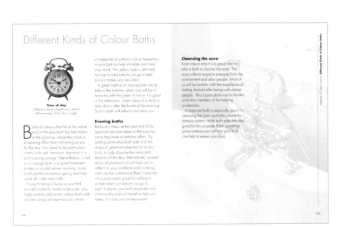

Detail
In-depth spreads provide further information and detail.

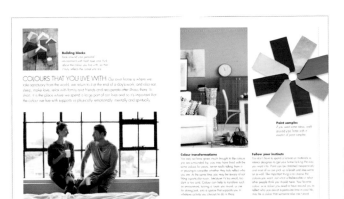

Environment
Learn how the colours in your environment, including clothes and interiors, can help enhance your mental well-being.

Introduction

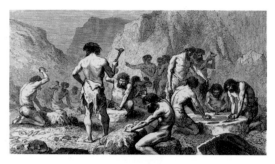

Survival
Colour has played a vital part in human health, survival and culture since ancient times.

Colour is, quite simply, light and none of us can live without it. The cells of our bodies react to it, or the lack of it, and this affects directly our physical, emotional, mental and spiritual well-being. We have only to think of how we intuitively respond to colour – such as with awe at the splendour of a sunrise, or with hope at the magic of a rainbow – to realize its power to heal.

The first colour healers

Our primitive ancestors were much more in touch with the healing properties of colour than we are today. From their observation of nature and the world around them, they learned to attribute certain properties to certain colours and these properties still hold good today. For instance red was the colour of the precious fire that warmed their bodies and over which they cooked their food; it was also the colour of the blood that ran through their veins. Red was therefore the colour of life and so figured prominently in their art and rituals.

Dyes & pigments

Dark blue, or indigo, was the colour of the sky under which they slept at night and dreamed to awake refreshed to another day. And green was the colour of the wild plants that they sought out for food or as medicine when they were sick or wounded.

Our ancestors also used colour in the form of natural dyes extracted from plants. This was employed to decorate their bodies. Pigments were also made from ground minerals or crushed berries and used to paint the walls of the caves in which they lived.

The colour of the environment

We too express ourselves through the colour we wear and the colours with which we decorate our home environment. We are also instinctively drawn to the particular colours that we require in order to correct an imbalance of energy in ourselves, which may be resulting in physical, mental or emotional problems. By eating, wearing or surrounding ourselves with the colour – exposing ourselves to it in some way – we heal ourselves. This is the very essence of colour healing and is part of the ancient wisdom that we have begun to return to in the New Age.

Electromagnetic Spectrum

White light is made up of many different colours, of which the human eye can only see about 40 per cent. Each colour has a different wavelength and vibrational frequency. The electromagnetic waves we cannot see are radio waves, infrared, ultraviolet, X-rays and gamma waves. Some people believe we are capable of seeing colours outside our normal range by using our 'third eye' (see page 37).

HISTORY OF
COLOUR HEALING

Colour healing has its roots in the ancient civilizations of Egypt, India and China, and even lost Atlantis. In the circular temples of Atlantis there are reputed to have been special chambers where people went to be healed by a combination of natural light and crystals. The temples of the ancient Egyptians were likewise constructed to channel the rays of the sun for healing purposes. The great cathedrals of the Middle Ages were similarly fitted with stained glass windows, through which the sun cast pools of coloured light in which the weak and sick could bathe and have their health restored. Humanity has always worshipped the sun – its light contains all the colours of the spectrum and has been known for its healing properties since ancient times.

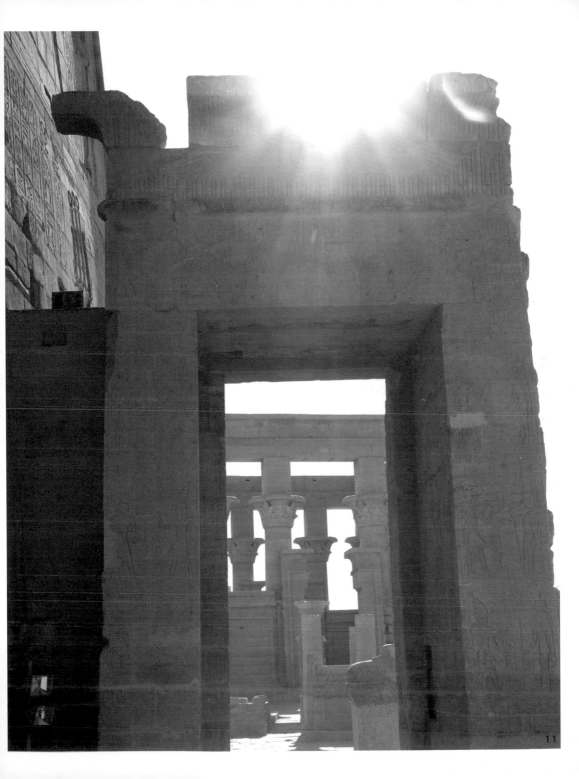

The Doctrine of Humours

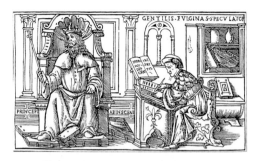

Colour treatment

The great physicians of ancient times, including Avicenna, used colour to treat the various ills of their patients.

Throughout the Middle Ages the treatment of disease, or imbalance in the body, was led by the *Doctrine of Humours*. According to this doctrine there were four main bodily fluids or humours – blood, phlegm, choler (bile) and black choler. These corresponded to the four astrological elements – Fire, Earth, Air and Water (see pages 30–33) – and were associated with the qualities of heat, dryness, coldness and moisture.

Each humour also related to a particular colour and constitution or temperament. Therefore, an excess of red blood meant that the person was considered to be of a sanguine or cheerful and optimistic disposition; if white phlegm was dominant, then the person was stolid in nature; yellow bile meant that the person was quick to anger or irascible; black bile denoted a person of melancholy disposition.

Avicenna

It was believed that if the humours were out of proportion to one another in the body, treatment using the relevant colour (see below) could bring them back into balance.

This type of colour therapy was known to physicians of ancient times too; the Persian physician, Avicenna (980–1037), wrote in his influential *Canon of Medicine* that red stimulated the circulation of the blood. So, someone who was bleeding should not look at anything red; rather he or she should look upon blue because it had a calming effect, reducing the flow of blood. Accordingly, he prescribed (inspired by the work of great philosophers and physicians such as Aristotle, Pythagoras and Hippocrates) coloured ointments, bandages and flowers in his treatment of disease.

Paracelsus

One of the best-known physicians of the Renaissance period was a Swiss who called himself Paracelsus (1493–1541). He was a man possessed of remarkable healing talents and used colour in his treatment of patients. He also used herbs, music and many of the other alternative or complementary medicines that are gaining in popularity today. However, his name meant 'greater than Celsus', the famous physician of ancient Rome, and his outspoken attitude to the authorities of the day made him many enemies. During his lifetime his work was not given the recognition it deserved.

Hippocrates

Hippocrates (c. 460–c. 377 BCE) defined man according to the four elements, relating male to Fire (red) and Air (yellow), female to Earth (green) and Water (blue).

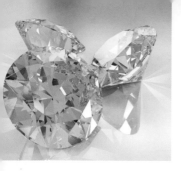

Crystal light
A crystal refracts light into the colours of the spectrum in much the same way as a prism.

DISCOVERING COLOUR

The great English mathematician and physicist, Sir Isaac Newton (1642–1727) is best known for his formulation of the laws of gravity, but he also discovered how the colour spectrum is produced. This discovery came about quite accidentally when Cambridge University was closed down during the Great Plague and he was forced to continue his studies at home. Newton's work forms the basis of today's understanding of colour.

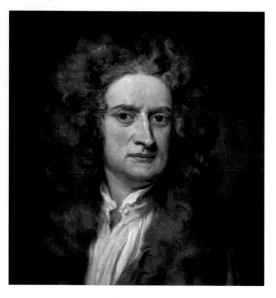

Newton
Newton's scientific theory of refraction is spectacularly demonstrated in nature by the phenomenon of the rainbow.

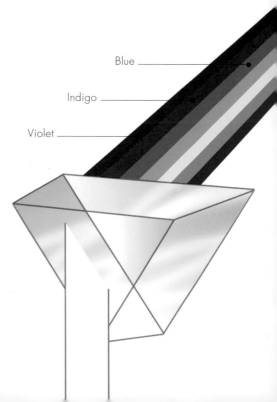

Blue

Indigo

Violet

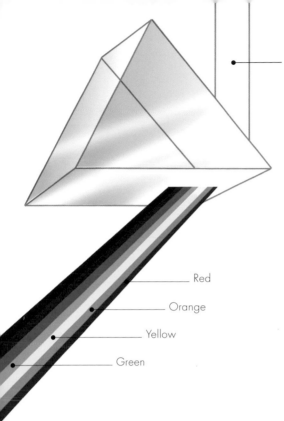

White light is refracted, forming the spectrum of seven colours, when it passes through a prism

Red

Orange

Yellow

Green

Newton's prism

While working at home on understanding the nature of light, Newton experimented with passing the sunlight that entered his room through a prism. It was then that he discovered that the light was refracted or deflected into the colours of the spectrum.

When he experimented further, he found that each colour had a different angle of refraction and this is what made it visible to the human eye as red, orange, yellow and so on. He also found that if he turned the prism upside down, the colours combined to form white light again.

Newton concluded that light, or colour, consists of waves, and each colour has a different wavelength and vibrates at a different frequency. This is how he arrived at what we now know is the scientific explanation of colour.

D.P. Ghadiali

It was a Hindu scientist, D.P. Ghadiali (1873–1966), working in the United States in the early part of the twentieth century, who formulated the scientific principles behind the effects the different colours have on the human body. He found that for each organism or system there was a particular colour that stimulated, and another that inhibited, its functioning. It therefore followed that if a part of the body was not functioning normally, balance could be restored by treatment with the appropriate colour.

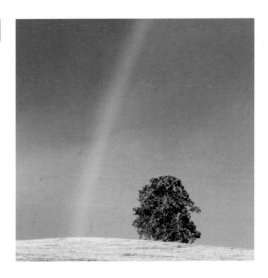

Edwin Babbitt
& Rudolf Steiner

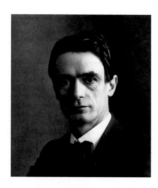

Steiner
Rudolf Steiner's ideas on colour are still used in schools today to encourage children to learn.

One of the most important pioneers of colour healing was the American Edwin D. Babbitt (1828–1905). His magnum opus, *The Principles of Light and Colour*, caused quite a stir when published in 1878. In his book Babbitt described the different healing effects of the colours of the spectrum and identified red as stimulating the blood, blue as calming it and orange and yellow as useful for stimulating the nerves. Accordingly, Babbitt prescribed treatment with red for paralysis; blue for inflammatory and nervous conditions; and yellow to act as a laxative.

Babbitt invented various devices for treatment with colour including the Chromalume, a kind of cabinet in which the patient sat, exposed to the light of the sun, in order to be bathed in colour from a window made of coloured glass. Many of Babbitt's devices were originally banned, but still served as prototypes for aids to colour treatment that are used today.

Rudolf Steiner

The Austrian philosopher, mystic and educationist, Rudolf Steiner (1861–1925), used colour in his spiritual teachings. Although educated as a scientist, from an early age Steiner experienced a spiritual reality that could not be explained in terms of the material world. Later he founded Anthroposophy, a movement that seeks to develop people's spiritual perception and understanding of themselves in relation to the universe. This led to the founding of Steiner schools.

Steiner's first centre for spiritual learning, the *Goetheanum* in Dornach, in Switzerland, had coloured glass windows to help people become aware of the different effects of colour. Blue brought a sense of peace, green a feeling of harmony, violet enhanced self-respect and rose gave rise to feelings of unconditional love. In Steiner schools today, this use of colour is reflected at every stage of a child's development, with bright, warm colours for the young and cooler colours for older children.

Steiner & Goethe

Steiner was influenced by J.W. von Goethe (1749–1832), the great German writer. Goethe mounted a crusade against Newton and his scientific theory of colour (see pages 14–15), arguing that colours were seen by the eye according to prevailing conditions and were a combination of light and darkness. Goethe's theory did not convince scientists.

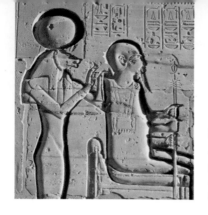

Healing gods
Ancient gods and goddesses of healing have inspired the colour therapists of today.

THEO GIMBEL
Described as the elder statesman of modern colour therapy, particularly in Britain, Gimbel has been much influenced by the work of Goethe and Steiner. However, he has formulated his own unique approach to colour therapy, following on from ancient esoteric teachings.

Colour pioneer

It was Gimbel's experiences as a prisoner of war in Russia, and later as a teacher of mentally handicapped children, that led him to develop a lifelong interest in the effects of colour. After many years of research, he founded the Hygeia College of Colour Therapy, which was named, appropriately, after the Greek goddess of health. At this college Gimbel has trained many of the colour therapists practising today. Gimbel was influenced by Goethe and this picture shows a table of colour refraction from one of Goethe's works on colour: *Zur Farbenlehre.*

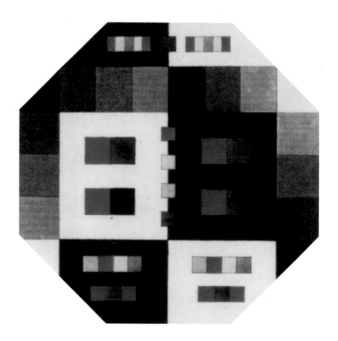

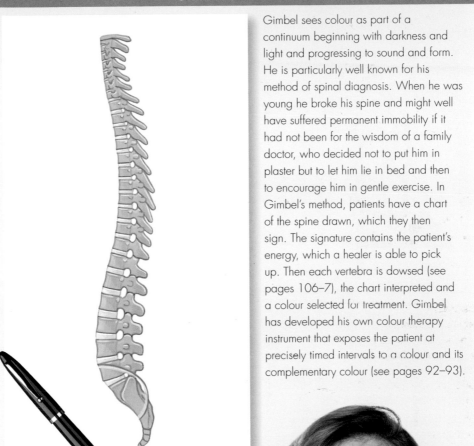

Gimbel sees colour as part of a continuum beginning with darkness and light and progressing to sound and form. He is particularly well known for his method of spinal diagnosis. When he was young he broke his spine and might well have suffered permanent immobility if it had not been for the wisdom of a family doctor, who decided not to put him in plaster but to let him lie in bed and then to encourage him in gentle exercise. In Gimbel's method, patients have a chart of the spine drawn, which they then sign. The signature contains the patient's energy, which a healer is able to pick up. Then each vertebra is dowsed (see pages 106–7), the chart interpreted and a colour selected for treatment. Gimbel has developed his own colour therapy instrument that exposes the patient at precisely timed intervals to a colour and its complementary colour (see pages 92–93).

Spinal diagnosis

Using Gimbel's method the patient signs a drawing of his or her spine. Then each vertebra is dowsed to find the appropriate colour for treatment.

Modern Applications of Colour

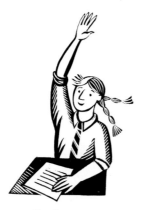

Environment
Colour is used in different environments, including schools, to influence people to behave in certain ways.

The work of the pioneers in colour healing was overshadowed by scientific and technological advances in modern medicine. But while modern medicine has long used the colours at the invisible end of the colour spectrum, infrared and ultraviolet, it is only relatively recently that medical practitioners have begun to use the visible colours. Blue light, in particular, has been shown to be effective in the treatment of various diseases, both physical and psychological, including cancer, eating disorders and various addictions.

Generally speaking, the medical profession has become more aware of the physical and psychological effects of colour. This can be seen, for example, in the choice of colour for gowns worn in hospital operating theatres: green for harmony, or light blue for calmness and coolness.

Mood shifters

Other professions and institutions, such as prisons and schools, also consciously use certain colours. In prisons, the use of soft pink to paint walls has been shown to reduce the incidence of aggressive and violent behaviour in inmates; while in schools yellow has been shown to stimulate learning. However, yellow is a colour to be avoided in the environment of the mentally ill or highly stressed because it is possible that it will overexcite sufferers.

Artificial light

Natural light is beneficial to us, but some artificial light has been shown to have a detrimental effect on people exposed to it, whether in the office or in public places. For example, some people react adversely to fluorescent light because it is lacking in the colours at the blue end of the spectrum and has a fast flicker. It has been shown to cause headaches and stress.

Photobiologist Dr John Ott developed the full-spectrum tube that is in use in many offices today. This provides a close equivalent of daylight and is therefore much healthier.

Theo Gimbel (see pages 18–19) has done extensive research into sodium street lighting, showing that it creates a negative environment that can lead to depression and crime. He advocates the installation of street lighting that is made up of light toward the blue end of the spectrum, in order to reduce stress and violent behaviour.

COLOURS OF THE SPECTRUM

Light, more specifically the colours that are visible to the human eye, actually occupies only a small part of the electromagnetic spectrum. This spectrum includes infrared light at one end and ultraviolet light at the other, which we cannot see. It also includes X-rays, gamma rays, radio waves and microwaves; the latter two are so-called because, like the rest of the spectrum, this kind of energy radiates out in waves. The distance from one crest of a wave to another – known as the wavelength – determines what kind of wave it is. The wavelength varies depending on the colour, the longest being at the red end and the shortest at the violet end. These seven colours – red, orange, yellow, green, blue, indigo and violet – are also known as the seven rays.

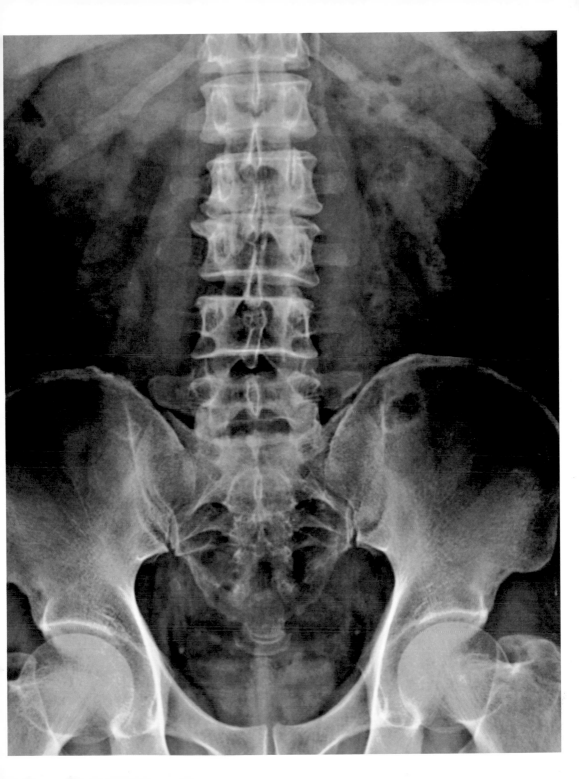

How We React to Colour

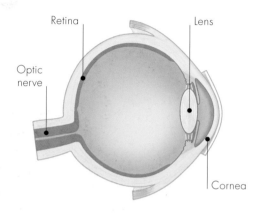

Retina

Lens

Optic
nerve

Cornea

The eye
*Light enters our bodies through the
eye, where the light-sensitive retina
breaks it down into colour.*

Just as the colours of the spectrum
can be produced by directing
sunlight through a prism (see pages
14–15), so a rainbow is created when
the rays of the sun are refracted through
drops of rain. The larger the drops,
the brighter the colours.

The lens of the eye similarly acts to
refract or change the direction of light,
focusing it on the retina, which is the light-
sensitive membrane found at the back
of the eye. There the light then stimulates
two kinds of cells, known as rod cells and
cone cells. Rod cells are sensitive to
dim light, enabling us to distinguish
between light and shade, and day and
night, while cone cells are sensitive to the
wavelengths of the three primary colours,
red, green and blue. When light hits
these cells it triggers nerve impulses that
are transmitted via the optic nerve to the
brain, where the image is then formed.
And that is how we see colour.

Colour, hormones & behaviour

Colour produces a biochemical reaction
within our bodies, directly stimulating
important glands, like the pituitary gland
for instance, which is the master gland
of the endocrine system. This gland
produces the hormones that regulate
our bodily functions – our sleep patterns,
sex drive, metabolic rate, appetite and
so on – as well as our moods, emotions
and behaviour. Two of the most important
hormones are melatonin and serotonin,
and these are both secreted by the pineal
gland, which is located in the brain.
The production of serotonin is stimulated
by day and the production of melatonin

by night. Serotonin has an uplifting effect, helping us to stay awake and be alert, while melatonin has a sedative effect, aiding sleep.

SAD

High levels of melatonin have been found in people suffering from SAD, or Seasonal Affective Disorder. This is a specific type of depression that many people suffer from in the winter months due to lack of sunlight. Some of the symptoms include the desire to sleep, general fatigue and a lack of interest in sex. However, such people have been found to respond dramatically to treatment with full-spectrum white light.

Genetic Programming

This direct response to the lack of colour in winter is thought to be held deep in our genetic memory. This goes back to the time when, like animals, we hibernated in winter due to the necessity to survive when the weather was extreme and food was scarce.

Nec species sua cuique manet, rerumque novatrix
ex aliis alias reddit natura figuras.
nec perit in toto quidquam, mihi credite, mundo,
sed variat faciemque novat, nascique vocatur
incipere esse aliud, quam quod fuit ante, morique,
desinere illud idem. Cum sint huc forsitan illa,
haec translata illuc, summa tamen omnia constant.

Purple prose

*'Purple prose' describes
flowery language in which
the writer gets carried away.*

THE PSYCHOLOGY OF COLOUR
The profound effect colour has on our moods, emotions and behaviour is reflected in the sayings that pepper our everyday language. We unconsciously resort to these to describe how we are feeling or to explain our reaction to something. Using colours that everyone can relate to in these sayings makes them an extremely effective form of communication.

Green with envy

To be 'green with jealousy or envy' is to be emotionally out of balance – green is the colour that holds the balance between the warm or red end of the colour spectrum and the cool or blue end.

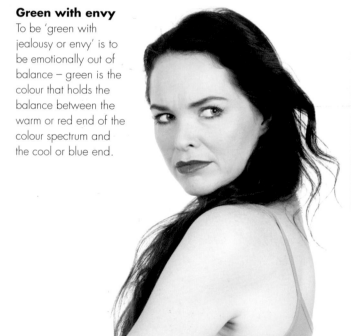

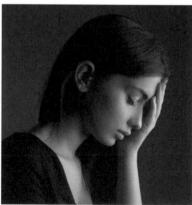

The blues

When we say we have 'the blues', we are communicating that we are in solitary, introverted mode.

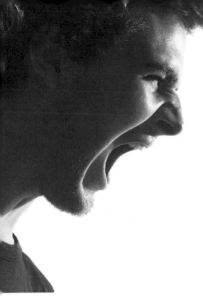

Seeing red

When we say we 'see red' or 'it was like
a red rag to a bull', we are describing
a response that is invariably immediate
and involves anger or aggression. This is
something that is very deeply ingrained in
us. If our ancestors had not met the threat of
danger with the will to fight or the strength
and speed to run away – the so-called
'fight or flight' response – we would not
have evolved to the present day.

Black dog

A 'colourful character' is someone who has
lived a full and interesting life; 'colourful language'
often includes words of the four-letter variety into which
a lot of physical energy is usually put. By contrast,
we talk about the 'black dog' of depression, using
black to describe a world from which all
colour, or life, seems to have disappeared.

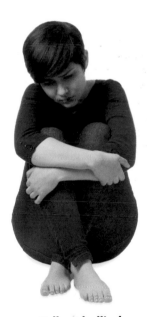

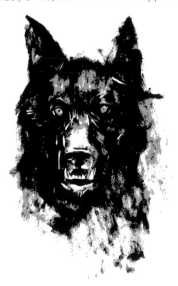

Yellow-bellied

'Yellow' or 'yellow-bellied' is often
used to describe a coward, someone
who will not move to defend him-
or herself or someone else.

Colour & Personality

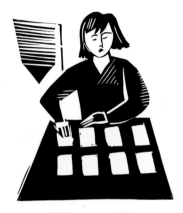

Colour you like
The colours that you choose say a lot about the kind of person you are and what you like.

We all have preferences for one colour or another and these colours say a lot about us, psychologically as well as physically. A Swiss professor of psychology, Max Lüscher, is famous for developing a test for analysing people's colour preferences according to their personality type.

In the Lüscher Colour Test, people were asked to select a range of colours in order of preference. Someone who chose red was likely to be assertive or aggressive, strong-willed and confident, of the 'red' personality type; on the other hand, someone who chose blue was likely to be shy or usually held themselves aloof, of the 'blue' personality type.

There is now some controversy over the colours Lüscher chose for his test – he included brown, grey and black, which are not colours of the spectrum – and other, more modern tests have since been devised. It is also true to say that a red personality type, someone with high blood pressure, say, or a quick temper, is just as likely to avoid the colour and opt for its cooling opposite, blue, instead. The colours we like are often the colours we instinctively know we need.

Colour is personal

Our choice of colour is intensely personal; the clothes we wear, the decor of our homes, even the car we drive, are all making personal statements about ourselves. When we decide to change our colour scheme – paint a room a different colour, or wear a different colour – we are saying something different about ourselves, whether we know it or not.

It is important to wear, or have around you, the colours you like – they will have a positive effect on you. A colour may have a special meaning for you because it is associated with a happy memory, perhaps from childhood. If you live in the city now, for example, but were brought up in the country, you may long for the sight of green fields. A walk in the countryside may be just what you need to refresh yourself after the stress of city life. Or, failing that, try hanging pictures of landscapes on the walls in which the colour green predominates.

Dowsing for Colour

If you are not sure what colour you need in your life right now, try dowsing to find out (see pages 106–7). Once you know, you will discover that you start attracting it to yourself – it will suddenly leap out at you, in the dress or shirt that someone is wearing, in an advertisement on a billboard or even in a certain fruit on a market stall.

ASTROLOGY & COLOUR

There are 12 signs of the zodiac; the Sun, the Moon and 8 planets; and 4 elements (Fire, Earth, Air and Water). Fire is associated with the colour red, Earth with green, Water with blue and Air with yellow. The signs of the zodiac are divided into Fire, Earth, Air or Water signs (see pages 32–33). The Sun, Moon and planets are positioned in the signs. An astrologer can calculate your birthchart and discover what you have in the signs or elements, in order to determine which colours dominate and which are lacking.

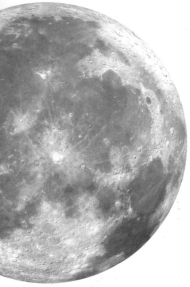

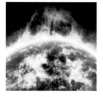

The Sun
The masculine or active energy, the Sun is a bright golden yellow, a hot and fierce energy that it is dangerous to expose yourself to for too long.

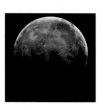

Mercury
The planet of the mind and communication, is usually depicted as yellow, the colour of the intellect.

Mars
The planet of action, aggression and war, is an unequivocal red.

MOON

MARS

The Moon
On the other hand, the Moon is the feminine or receptive energy. It is a silvery white, and in its radiance we can seek to escape the everyday world and aspire to a different kind of reality.

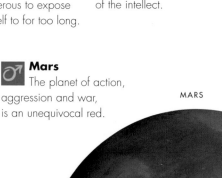

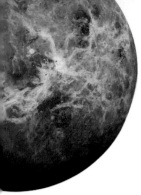

VENUS

The most important of the ten heavenly bodies are the Sun and the Moon, also known as the Lights or Luminaries.

In addition to the planets Mercury, Venus and Mars, in ancient or traditional astrology there were two more planets: Jupiter and Saturn.

Modern astrology has added three more planets, discovered recently: Uranus, Neptune and the dwarf planet Pluto.

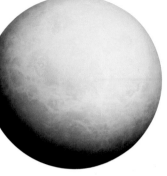

URANUS

Venus
The planet of love, beauty and the arts, Venus is green, which is the colour of growth, fecundity and balance.

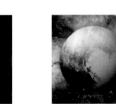

Jupiter
The planet of expansion and good fortune, is purple.

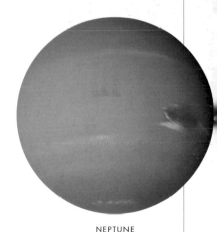

Pluto
This dwarf planet controls all the things we do not want to know about – repressed emotions, dark secrets and compulsions – and is, of course, black.

Uranus
This planet rules new ideas, especially those that challenge the status quo, and is sky blue.

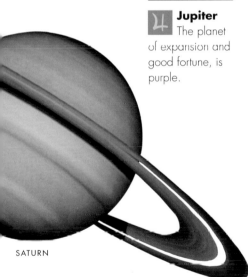

SATURN

Saturn
The planet of work, responsibility and duty, which, appropriately, is brown or black.

NEPTUNE

Neptune
This planet rules all things watery, emotional and spiritual, and is, as you would expect, a deep blue.

The Elements

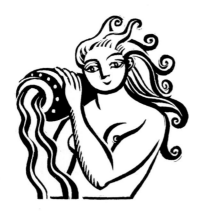

Planets
*The number of planets you
have in the elements tells you
what colour you lack.*

The 12 signs of the zodiac fall into four groups of three, which are divided by the elements:
• **The Fire signs** Aries, Leo and Sagittarius.
• **The Earth signs** Taurus, Virgo and Capricorn.
• **The Air signs** Gemini, Libra and Aquarius.
• **The Water signs** Cancer, Pisces and Scorpio.

Each of these groups has its own distinguishing characteristics, both negative and positive. The Fire signs are noted for their energy, spontaneity, intuition and

belief in themselves, but they can also be egotistical and overbearing. If your birthchart shows that you have a lot of planets in Fire, you have a lot of red energy.

The Earth signs tend to be sensual, productive, conservative and grounded in the material world. However, they can also be unimaginative and narrow-minded. If you have a lot of planets in the Earth element, you have a lot of green energy.

The Air signs are intelligent, sociable, communicative and at home in the world of ideas; they can also be malicious and unfeeling. If you have a lot of planets in Air, then you have a lot of yellow energy.

The Water signs are sensitive, emotional, imaginative and need to experience a soul or spiritual connection with others. However, they also tend to be melodramatic and irrational. If you have a lot of planets in Water, then you have a lot of blue energy.

The missing element
It is quite common to have very few planets, or even none at all, in one of the elements, which then becomes your missing element. For example, if you have no planets in Fire, then that means

that you are lacking red energy; if you have no planets in Water, then you are lacking blue energy.

You can also have an excess of certain elements. If you have a 'red' planet like Mars in one of the Fire signs, it can give you an excess of red energy, while having a lot of the planets in the Air signs can give you an excess of yellow energy.

Once you have all this vital information you can then choose to surround yourself with the colours you need to balance your energies.

Astrology

Astrology links the movements of the planets to events on Earth, allowing the astrologer to predict what is likely to happen in a person's life. The signs of the zodiac relate to the twelve 30° sectors in the Sun's annual path.

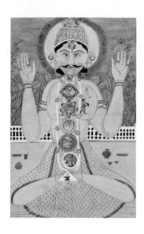

Balance of colour
Being healthy means balancing the colour energies of different parts of the body.

THE SEVEN RAYS These are the seven visible colours of the spectrum – red, orange, yellow, green, blue, indigo and violet. The seven rays correspond to the seven chakras or energy centres in the body (see pages 100–1). On a spiritual level, they symbolize great cosmic forces that represent different evolutionary stages in the history of humanity.

Evolution
We are currently thought to be evolving from the red end of the spectrum to the blue end, which is associated more with the higher manifestation of our being. It is interesting to note in this respect to our growing concern with green or environmental issues and the growth of the ecological movement and political parties concerned with green issues.

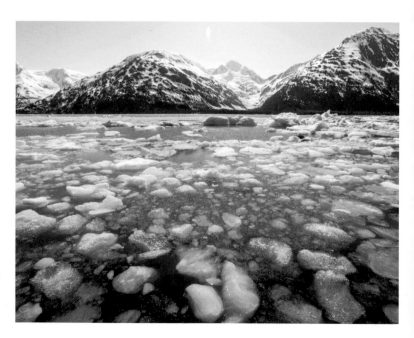

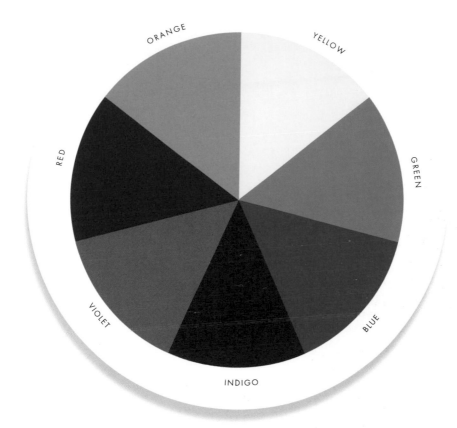

Qualities of the rays

The seven rays are also associated with different qualities, which we all have to a greater or lesser degree. A few people are only of one ray and they are then said to be 'on' the blue ray or whatever; most of us are a mixture of rays.

Ray Qualities		
Colour	**Positive**	**Negative**
Red	Strength	Brutality
Orange	Acceptance	Indifference
Yellow	Intellect	Coldness
Green	Empathy	Self-absorption
Blue	Justice	Intolerance
Indigo	Devotion	Self-delusion
Violet	Mysticism	Arrogance

Properties of the Rays

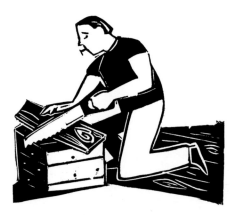

Type of person
The colour of the energy you have helps to define what type of person you are both physically and psychologically.

The rays have both physical and psychological attributes. Those at the red or warm end of the spectrum are more physical, and reflect the way in which we express ourselves outwardly, while those at the blue or cool end are more psychological, and echo our inner selves.

The warm rays

The red ray correlates with the base chakra at the root of the spine and this stimulates our physical vitality, which is particularly important for the procreative functions of the body. It is also associated with the qualities of strength, will and courage.

The orange ray helps the assimilative and digestive processes of the body and it relates to the second or navel chakra. People with a lot of orange energy are healthy in mind and body, always think positively and are physically active.

Yellow is the ray of the intellect and its chakra is situated at the solar plexus, an important centre for the nervous system. The yellow ray is associated with the qualities of intelligence, rationality and the ability to concentrate and focus.

Green is in the middle of the spectrum and is the colour of the heart chakra in the middle of the chest. This is the ray of harmony and balance, sympathy, compassion and devotion.

The cool rays

Blue is the first of the cool colours of the spectrum, and these rays counter or slow down the warm colours. This end of the spectrum takes us inwards and upwards, away from the physical and toward the spiritual. Blue relates to the throat chakra – the centre of speech – and its qualities are truth, sincerity and reflectiveness.

The indigo ray takes us higher still, into the realms controlled by the brow chakra, or third eye. This enables us to see in the psychic sense, discerning things not perceived by the five senses. The qualities of this ray are vision, inspiration and service to humanity.

Violet is the last of the colours of the spectrum and people on this ray are at a high level of consciousness. It is the ray of the crown chakra, situated on top of the head, and its qualities are spirituality, mysticism and the expression of the higher self.

Chakras & Colour Healing

Chakras are energy centres in the body, and if they are not functioning properly, they can detrimentally affect well-being. Each chakra is associated with a colour, so any imbalance should be treated using the relevant colour.

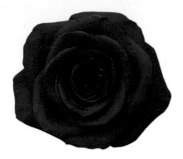

Red rose
A red rose symbolizes passion and is habitually given to the one we love.

RED Red is the colour of life itself, of fire and of blood, of danger and sex, and without it our lives would lack vigour, warmth, strength and passion. We need it in the food we eat, the clothes we wear and our physical surroundings in order to stimulate our nervous system, release adrenaline into the blood and improve our circulation. We also need red to root ourselves in everyday reality and to give us a sense of security.

A red rag to a bull
Red is a very physical colour and often provokes a physical reaction, sometimes violent.

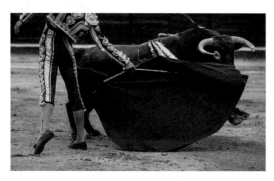

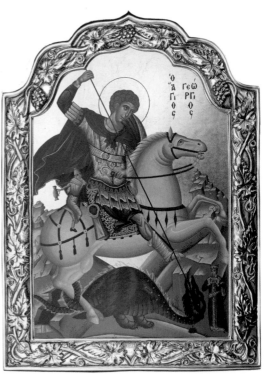

Saint George
St George slaying the dragon illustrates the strength, courage and aggression that are associated with red.

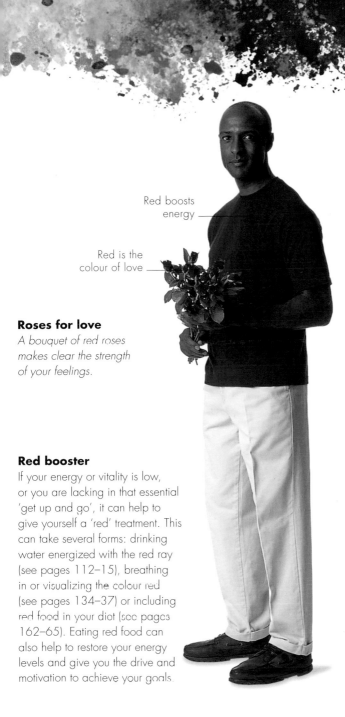

Red boosts energy

Red is the colour of love

Roses for love

A bouquet of red roses makes clear the strength of your feelings.

Red booster

If your energy or vitality is low, or you are lacking in that essential 'get up and go', it can help to give yourself a 'red' treatment. This can take several forms: drinking water energized with the red ray (see pages 112–15), breathing in or visualizing the colour red (see pages 134–37) or including red food in your diet (see pages 162–65). Eating red food can also help to restore your energy levels and give you the drive and motivation to achieve your goals.

(see pages 92–93).

Caution

Red is a very powerful colour and should not be used if you suffer from high blood pressure or heart problems, have a quick temper or are feeling angry or upset because it will only overstimulate you. You should also be aware that treatment with red should always be complemented by treatment with blue or green (see pages 92–93).

Healing with Red

Treatment with red can benefit the following conditions:

PHYSICAL CONDITIONS

low energy

anaemia

poor circulation

low blood pressure

colds/chills

NEGATIVE STATES OF MIND

apathy

depression

fear

lack of confidence/initiative

Using the Colour Red

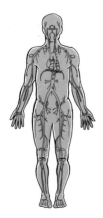

Lifeblood
*Red is the colour of the lifeblood
that flows through our veins and
circulates round our bodies.*

Red is the colour of the element of
Fire, the element of the signs of the
zodiac Aries, Leo and Sagittarius
(see pages 32–33) and is particularly
associated with the planet Mars, which
is known as 'the red planet'. Mars rules
aggression and sex drive and the part
of the body that the colour red relates
to is the genitals. It is therefore a good
colour to wear if your libido is low or
you want to spice up your sex life.

One of the main attributes of the colour
red is passion, the zest for life as well
as sexual passion. We give red roses to
the one we love, and Valentine's Day is
characterized by a flurry of red hearts
on cards and giftware. In this context,
too, red can also be a euphemism – an
insalubrious part of a town is usually
known as 'the red-light district'.

People on the red ray, or those with
a lot of red energy, tend to be positive,
confident and optimistic about the future.
They usually look forward to the day
ahead and face obstacles with courage
and strength. However, they can also
express their 'red' traits more negatively,
by selfishly pursuing their own ends
without regard for the feelings of others.

Affirmations

If you are feeling at a low ebb, either
physically or emotionally, and want
to give yourself a boost, it can help
to practise one of the colour healing
treatments described on pages 38–39.

You can also write yourself a 'red'
affirmation. Affirmations are simple
sentences, best written in the present
tense, which affirm or positively reinforce
a state of being. They can be spoken
while looking into a mirror, so that
the words are reflected back at you,

increasing their power and helping you
to absorb and act on your affirmation.
Alternatively, the words can be written
down on a piece of paper and put under
your pillow when you go to bed at night.
   If you repeat your affirmation often
enough, or continue to keep the piece
of paper under your pillow night after
night, your subconscious mind is likely
to receive the message it contains and
will react accordingly.

Red Qualities

Positive energetic, enthusiastic, assertive,
spontaneous, strong-willed, courageous, self-
motivated

Negative insensitive, aggressive, impatient,
domineering, self-centred

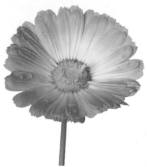

Marigold
*The daisy-like flowers of the
marigold cannot fail to cheer.*

ORANGE On the colour wheel, orange falls between red and yellow and it
therefore acts on both the physical body (red) and the intellect (yellow). Like red, it is
a strong and vibrant colour and needs to be used with care. We associate orange
with health and vitality. Many people start the day with a glass of orange juice, which
has a tonic effect and is full of the vitamin C that is needed to boost the immune system
and ward off colds and illnesses.

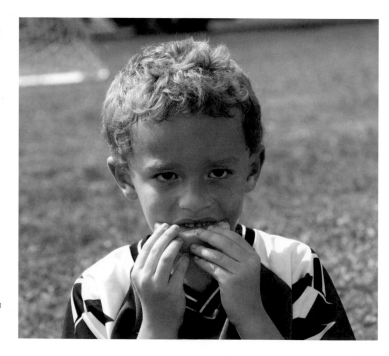

Youth & activity
*Orange is the colour of youth
and activity, and schoolchildren
are often given oranges to eat
at half-time during games.*

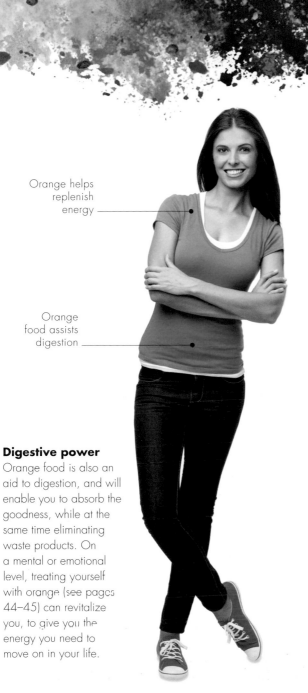

Orange helps
replenish
energy

Orange
food assists
digestion

Digestive power
Orange food is also an
aid to digestion, and will
enable you to absorb the
goodness, while at the
same time eliminating
waste products. On
a mental or emotional
level, treating yourself
with orange (see pages
44–45) can revitalize
you, to give you the
energy you need to
move on in your life.

(see pages 44–45)

Caution

You have no need of extra
orange if you are fit and well
and enjoying life. Too much
orange and you may become
complacent or self-indulgent. Like
red, orange is a strong colour
and needs to be used with care.

Healing with Orange

Treatment with orange can
benefit the following conditions:

PHYSICAL CONDITIONS

low vitality/appetite

indigestion

asthma

cramps

gallstones

NEGATIVE STATES OF MIND

listlessness

bereavement

inhibition

sadness

boredom

Using the Colour Orange

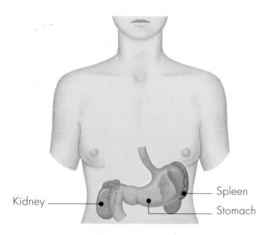

Kidney ——————

—————— Spleen

—————— Stomach

Digestive organs
*The colour orange is associated
with the digestive and eliminative
organs of the body.*

Orange relates to the spleen, an organ situated behind the stomach, on the left side of the abdomen. The spleen is connected both to the stomach and the kidneys and its function is to maintain the blood, keeping it clean and healthy. The spleen breaks up worn-out red and white blood cells and also stores red blood cells for use in emergencies.

The archaic meaning of 'spleen' is 'the seat of the emotions'. To 'vent one's spleen' is to be spiteful or disagreeable in some way. And just as the organ filters out impurities from the blood, so treatment with the colour orange can help you to assimilate negative feelings or come to terms with traumatic events in your life, such as the loss of someone close or the break-up of a relationship.

Orange can also be of benefit when you feel that you are in a rut, stuck in your life and fearful of making the changes that will enable you to leave the past behind and go forward into the future. The action associated with this colour is expansion, the opening up of yourself to life, so that you can engage with it once more.

Positive thinking

Orange is also associated with positive thinking and motivation, which is why it is often used in advertising by businesses who want to encourage us to buy certain products.

Writing an 'orange' affirmation can help you to regain a sense of *joie de vivre*. It will act as a kind of mental 'pick-me-up' in much the same way as drinking a glass of orange juice or water charged with orange energy (see pages 112–15) revitalizes the physical body.

It can also help to wear something orange. It doesn't have to be a complete outfit; orange is a very bright colour and is therefore not suitable for everyone's skin tone, but a scarf or tie, or even a piece of amber or coral jewellery is enough to make a difference. Even a simple gesture like placing a vase of sunny marigolds or striking tiger lilies in your surroundings can help to lift your mood. Try it and see how well it works.

Orange Affirmation

'I have a healthy mind and body and enjoy life to the full'.

Orange Qualities

Positive exuberant, sensual, gregarious, good-humoured, playful, sporty

Negative overindulgent, lazy, dependent, unkind, superficial

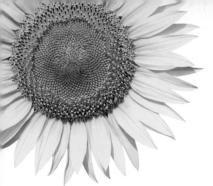

Yellow flowers
It's good to have yellow flowers in your environment if you are feeling depressed.

YELLOW

Perhaps more than any other flower, it is the daffodil that cheers us up after the long dark days of winter, its bright yellow trumpeting the arrival of spring. The poet William Wordsworth was so inspired by the sight of a bank of daffodils when he was out walking one day, that he wrote a poem about them. It begins with one of the most famous lines in the English language, 'I wandered lonely as a cloud'. In the poem Wordsworth speaks of how his spirits were lifted by the sight of the massed blooms, and continued to be, long after the moment had passed.

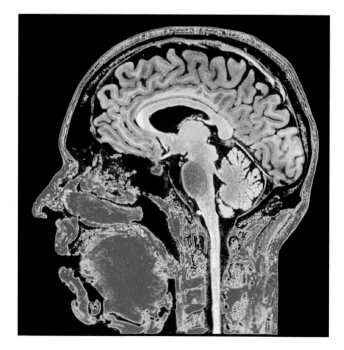

Left brain
The colour yellow relates to the rational mind and clear thinking, associated with the left brain, as opposed to intuition and clairvoyance, associated with the right brain.

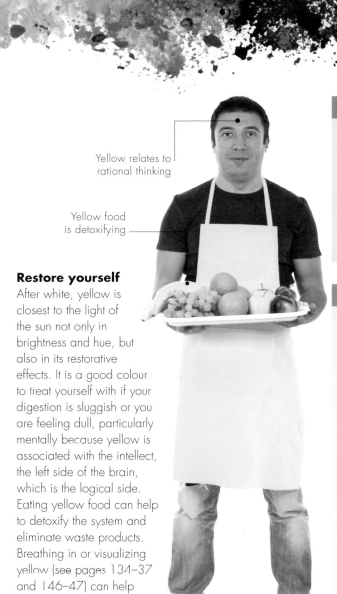

Yellow relates to
rational thinking

Yellow food
is detoxifying

Restore yourself

After white, yellow is
closest to the light of
the sun not only in
brightness and hue, but
also in its restorative
effects. It is a good colour
to treat yourself with if your
digestion is sluggish or you
are feeling dull, particularly
mentally because yellow is
associated with the intellect,
the left side of the brain,
which is the logical side.
Eating yellow food can help
to detoxify the system and
eliminate waste products.
Breathing in or visualizing
yellow (see pages 134–37
and 146–47) can help
you to focus mentally and
to concentrate on the task at
hand. It will also stimulate
the flow of ideas.

Healing with Yellow

Treatment with yellow can benefit
the following conditions:

PHYSICAL CONDITIONS

constipation

flatulence

diabetes

skin problems

nervous exhaustion

NEGATIVE STATES OF MIND

depression

low self-esteem

short attention span

examination nerves

writer's block

Using the Colour Yellow

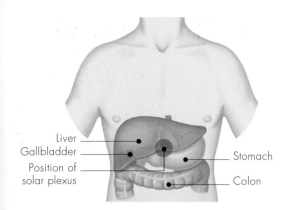

Liver
Gallbladder
Position of
solar plexus

Stomach

Colon

Solar plexus
Linked to the liver, intestines and gallbladder, the network of nerves that radiate out from the solar plexus resembles the rays of the sun.

Yellow relates to the solar plexus, the network of sympathetic nerves situated behind the stomach. It is linked to key abdominal organs: the liver, intestines and gallbladder.

The solar plexus is an important centre in the body for all the digestive processes and the word 'solar' comes from the Latin *sol*, which means 'sun' – the centre of the solar system.

Yellow stimulates the action of the abdominal organs – in particular the flow of bile, which plays an essential part in the digestion and absorption of fats. Bile is secreted by the liver, the chief function of which is to process what we eat into substances that the body needs.

In ancient times, the liver was considered to be the seat of love or passion, hence the expression 'lily-livered', to describe a coward.

Eliminating negativity

On a psychological, as well as physical, level yellow helps get things moving, eliminating negative thoughts and feelings that can undermine our sense of self-worth.

It can also do a similar thing in social circumstances; if you want your parties to be lively affairs, try introducing some yellow into the parts of your home where people gather. Too much, though, and people are likely to become overstimulated and start arguing with each other.

Yellow is also a good colour for children, since it helps to develop their cognitive abilities. If they have a playroom or study, it is beneficial to include some yellow in the room's colour scheme. It is wise to avoid painting children's bedrooms in this colour, however, because its stimulating qualities may cause restlessness and difficulty in sleeping.

The golden touch

Gold, or golden yellow, represents knowledge at its highest level; the wisdom gained through the assimilation of experience. In the spiritual sense this is ultimately more precious than the gold jewellery that is so often a symbol of wealth, status and privilege.

Yellow Qualities

Positive rational, clear thinking, broad-minded, detached, sociable

Negative critical, argumentative, opinionated, evasive, restless

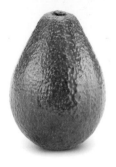

Green food
Green food is essential for good health, helping to keep our bodies in balance. Avocados are a good source of vitamins A and E.

GREEN
Green is the colour of nature – of the fields, hills and woods where we often go in order to refresh ourselves and recharge our batteries after a sojourn among the buildings of a town or city. In nature everything is in harmony and surrounded by it we can find our centre again after a busy, stressful time at work or with family.

Green Man
The Green Man is a potent symbol of the growth and fecundity of nature.

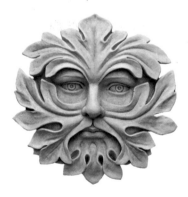

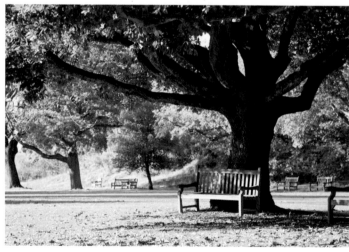

The soothing power of nature
If you are feeling out of sorts, it can often help to take a walk in the countryside; if that is not possible because you live in a town or city, you can always go to a park or public gardens. Do not be afraid to hug a tree, however ridiculous you think it may look; trees are great reservoirs of energy and can help to stabilize you if you are feeling fragile.

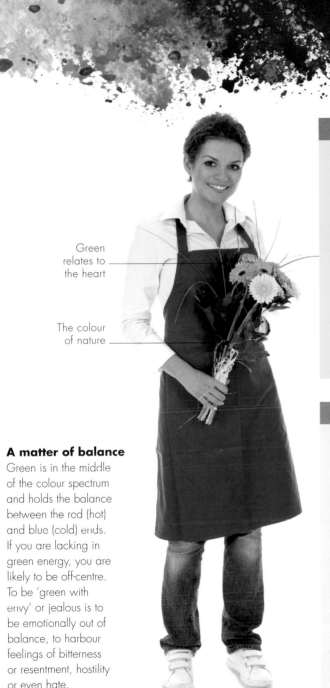

Green
relates to
the heart

The colour
of nature

Caution

Green is probably one of the safest colours of the spectrum. It is best avoided, however, in situations where you need to be mentally on the ball or are required to react quickly to what is happening, since it is such a good relaxer.

A matter of balance

Green is in the middle of the colour spectrum and holds the balance between the red (hot) and blue (cold) ends. If you are lacking in green energy, you are likely to be off-centre. To be 'green with envy' or jealous is to be emotionally out of balance, to harbour feelings of bitterness or resentment, hostility or even hate.

Healing with Green

Treatment with green can benefit the following conditions:

PHYSICAL CONDITIONS

heart problems

bronchitis

flu

claustrophobia

NEGATIVE STATES OF MIND

instability

brooding

fear of emotional involvement

spite

51

Using the Colour Green

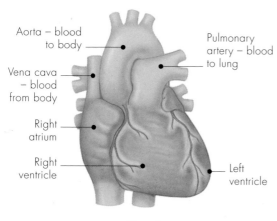

Aorta – blood to body

Pulmonary artery – blood to lung

Vena cava – blood from body

Right atrium

Right ventricle

Left ventricle

Heart

Just as green is the central colour of the spectrum, so the heart is the central organ of the body.

The part of the body that the colour green relates to is the heart, the muscular organ that pumps the lifeblood through our bodies. The heart is also the seat of the emotions, especially love, the most powerful emotion of all. The importance of this organ is reflected in the many sayings in which the word 'heart' appears.

If we 'break someone's heart', we cause someone deep emotional pain; when we 'lose heart' or say we 'haven't the heart' for something, we mean that we have no desire to do it, we cannot motivate ourselves. Similarly, when we speak 'from the bottom of our hearts', what we say is sincere, driven by profound emotion.

When two people have a 'heart to heart', they open up their hearts to each other – they hold nothing back, the emotions flow freely. Likewise, when we do something 'whole-heartedly', we give it everything we have got. Someone with a 'heart of gold' is a generous person, who will help someone else without thought of reward. In contrast, someone with a 'heart of stone' is cold, unfeeling and unlikely to answer a plea for help.

Heart attacks

It is generally accepted that heart attacks can often be caused by a deep-seated emotional problem, sometimes to do with a relationship. They may be brought on by repressing emotions, fear of emotional commitment or by being stuck in life and unable to change. Many men have heart attacks in middle age, which perhaps can be partly attributed to the fact that their heart is no longer in their career and gives out under the stress of the job.

Restorative power of green

One exercise you can do is to stand with your back against the trunk of a tree, then put your left arm out behind you around the tree, while holding your right hand over your solar plexus. Breathe in deeply, drawing the energy of the tree into yourself, then breathe out again. You will find that this will energize you and help to calm you down if you are feeling agitated.

Green Affirmation

'I am open to receiving everything that the universe has to give me'.

Green Qualities

Positive open, grounded, sympathetic, compassionate, generous, relaxed

Negative envious, mean, bitter, inflexible, jaded

53

Delphinium

The blue flowers of the delphinium are relaxing on the eye.

BLUE is the colour of the sky and the sea; looking up at a cloudless blue sky or gazing out at the sea can often still the mind and soothe the spirit. It is no coincidence that when we want to 'get away from it all', we often choose to take a holiday where we can gaze at limitless expanses of both sky and sea for hours on end, becoming so relaxed that we lose all sense of time passing.

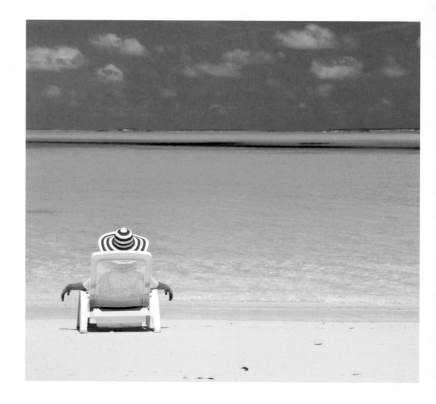

By the sea

A vacation by the sea helps us unwind and forget our cares.

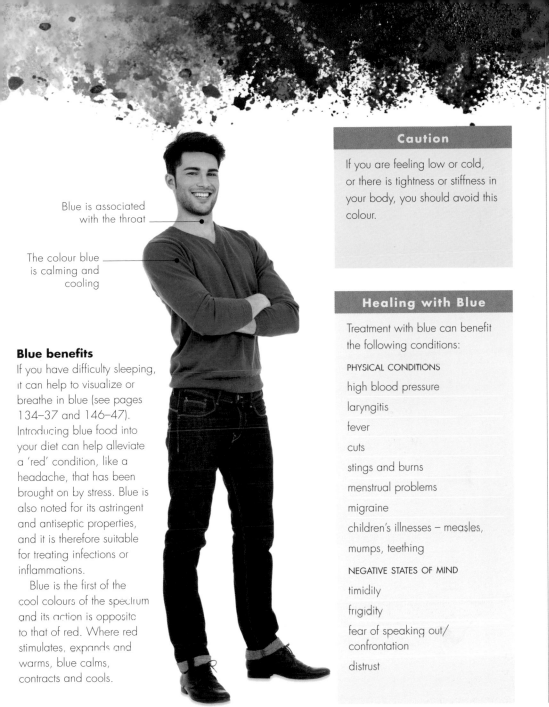

Blue is associated with the throat

The colour blue is calming and cooling

Blue benefits

If you have difficulty sleeping, it can help to visualize or breathe in blue (see pages 134–37 and 146–47). Introducing blue food into your diet can help alleviate a 'red' condition, like a headache, that has been brought on by stress. Blue is also noted for its astringent and antiseptic properties, and it is therefore suitable for treating infections or inflammations.

Blue is the first of the cool colours of the spectrum and its action is opposite to that of red. Where red stimulates, expands and warms, blue calms, contracts and cools.

Healing with Blue

Treatment with blue can benefit the following conditions:

PHYSICAL CONDITIONS

high blood pressure

laryngitis

fever

cuts

stings and burns

menstrual problems

migraine

children's illnesses – measles, mumps, teething

NEGATIVE STATES OF MIND

timidity

frigidity

fear of speaking out/confrontation

distrust

Using the Colour Blue

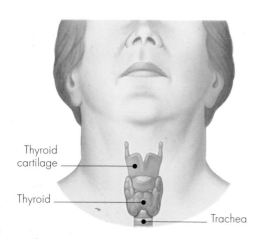

Thyroid cartilage

Thyroid

Trachea

Throat

Blue is associated with the throat and the power of speech, also wisdom.

The colour is associated with intelligence and the ability to speak your mind as well as to conciliate, or make peace, with words. Honesty and integrity are also 'blue' qualities; when we describe someone as 'true-blue', we mean we can count on them because they are loyal and trustworthy.

Speaking out

If you find it difficult to speak out, or cannot find your voice, it can help to treat yourself with blue. This may well clear the blockage, whether physical – in the form of a sore throat or hoarseness – or psychological, in the form of a terror of public speaking. Just wearing a blue scarf around your neck can help you overcome your fear. Singing in the shower can also do the same thing so it's a good place to practise using your voice.

The thyroid gland, which is the organ situated in the front of the neck connected to the larynx, is associated with the colour blue. The chief function of this gland is to produce the hormone controlling the body's rate of metabolism. It is one of the most important hormones in the human body; if it is deficient in children, they fail to grow and if it is deficient in adults, they become obese. Blue also governs the throat, which is the centre of speech, communication and self-expression.

With blue, the focus of our attention begins to shift inward, away from the physical world and toward the spiritual. It is the colour of contemplation and quiet reflection and a blue lamp or candle can be an aid to meditation (see pages 108–9). This will slow down the mind so that thoughts of a more inspirational nature may enter. Blue is also associated with writers, poets and philosophers.

Unfortunately, the 'blue' facility with words does have its negative side. The persuasiveness of 'blue' people, who are able to cajole you into doing what they want almost without your realizing it, can easily turn into manipulation. Similarly, in an attempt to avoid rows and confrontation, 'blue' people may unwittingly provoke dissent and argument.

Blue Affirmation

'I am at peace with myself and the world'.

Blue Qualities

Positive introspective, contemplative, serene, fluent, tactful, sincere, faithful

Negative tongue-tied, manipulative, disloyal, withdrawn, cold

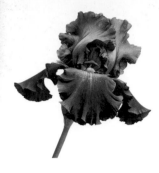

Iris
*The deep blue colour of indigo,
as seen in the iris flower, helps
free the imagination.*

INDIGO
Indigo is the colour of the sky at night – a deep, dark, velvety blue, both mysterious and unfathomable. When we gaze at it, our thoughts are likely to turn inward, causing us to ponder on the deeper meaning of life. At such times we are likely to have flashes of insight that do not come to us during the bright, busy, daylight hours.

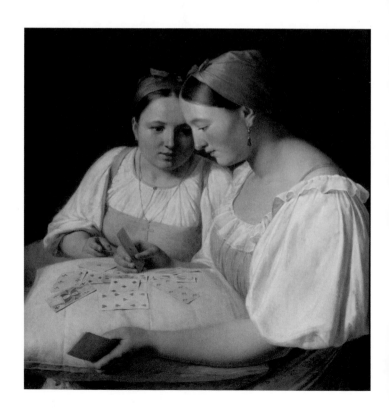

The fortune-teller
*The fortune-teller is inspired by
the intuitive colour of indigo to
give insights into the future.*

Indigo is
associated with
the brow chakra

Indigo relates
to intuition

Psychic power

Indigo purifies the mind, as
well as the blood. It frees us
of the fears and anxieties that
inhibit us to allow us to hear
our inner voice, which knows
what is best for us. If you
want to develop your psychic
potential, it is a good idea
to treat yourself with indigo,
visualizing the colour or
meditating on it (see pages
140–41 and 146–47).
It will lift you onto a higher
plane to enable you to see
with the inner eye. The insights
of indigo can also help with
deciphering the meaning
of dreams.

 Like all the colours at the blue
end of the spectrum, indigo helps
to take us away from the world
of the mundane, to more spiritual
dimensions, where intuition is
more important than reason and
faith more important than proof.

Healing with Indigo

Treatment with indigo can benefit
the following conditions:

PHYSICAL CONDITIONS

deafness

cataract

haemorrhage

nerves

NEGATIVE STATES OF MIND

obsession

paranoia

hysteria

over-sensitivity

Using the Colour Indigo

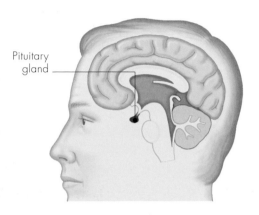

Pituitary gland

Master gland
The colour indigo is associated with the master gland of the body, which produces important hormones.

ndigo relates to the pituitary gland, which is situated at the base of the brain and is the most important endocrine gland in the body. It exerts overall control over other glands, including the thyroid and adrenal, through hormones it produces.

The colour indigo and the pituitary gland are associated in particular with the brow chakra, which is located between the eyebrows in the centre of the forehead. This area is perhaps better known as the third eye (see pages 36–37). This is the eye that sees what is invisible to the naked eye, far beyond the boundaries of time and space to other dimensions and realities. It is also known as the inner eye. When we talk of someone having 'the sight', we mean that they have this psychic or clairvoyant ability.

Inspiration
Someone with this ability can tap into a source of inspiration that gives people on this ray a reputation as spiritual teachers and healers. Going to a class or a talk given by such a person can act as a form of indigo treatment, helping to heal deep emotional hurts that have perhaps not been dealt with since childhood.

There are many such people around today, especially because humanity is evolving toward the blue end of the colour spectrum. More and more people report being able to see auras (coloured layers of light that emanate from the body – see pages 96–97), for example, or having dreams or visions that reveal their life path to them.

Helping others
Frequently such people develop the gifts of healing or psychic sensitivity, in order to be of service to their fellow human

beings. It is as if the third eye of humanity is collectively being opened at this time in history and we are all discovering that we have something to offer others.

However, on the negative side, 'indigo' people can become completely fanatical about things in which they believe, driven by a reforming zeal that is deaf to other people's points of view. This kind of blind devotion or prejudice can lead to intolerance and create division.

Indigo Affirmation

'I trust my intuition to guide me on my path through life'.

Indigo Qualities

Positive psychic, deep, visionary, wise, inspired

Negative fearful, arrogant, deluded, isolated, over-idealistic

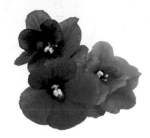

Glorious purple
The glorious purple of the violet helps take our mind away from everyday concerns.

VIOLET
The violet is a small and humble flower, yet to look upon a clump of them uplifts the spirits, and its sweet scent delights the senses. There is something noble about violet or purple and these colours have traditionally been worn by kings, clergy and those of high rank. In fact, at one time it was forbidden for lowlier folk to wear them.

Inspiration
In violet the blue colours of the spectrum reach their highest expression and this colour is associated with sacrifice, whether to a cause, ideal or to art. Violet is the colour of transcendence, of mind over matter and the higher self over the lower self. It is the colour of the divine inspiration, which is channelled by healer and artist alike.

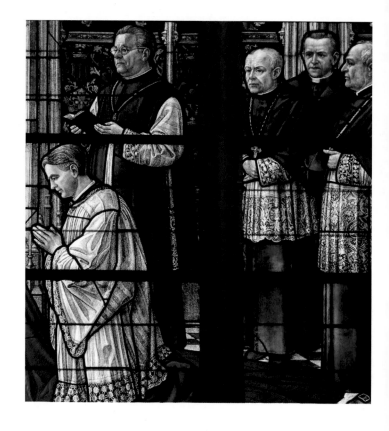

Noble purple
Throughout history violet or purple has been worn by royalty and senior clergy.

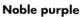

Violet contains
balancing energies ———

Violet is an
inspirational colour ———

Caution

Violet is a colour to be avoided
by people who suffer from
serious mental disorders or those
who have problems with alcohol
or drugs.

Meditative colour

If you are generally lacking in
inspiration, or you feel your life
lacks meaning, then violet is
a good colour to meditate on
(see pages 140–43), since it
helps to develop the psychic or
creative faculties. Meditating
on this colour may also help
you contact your spirit guides,
to obtain help in finding the
right direction for your life.
If you feel like retreating from
the world, or just want to take
things quietly, it can help to
switch to a diet containing
violet or purple food, as this
will calm you down and
nourish the spirit.

Healing with Violet

Treatment with violet can benefit
the following conditions:

PHYSICAL CONDITIONS

concussion

epilepsy

neuralgia

multiple sclerosis

NEGATIVE STATES OF MIND

neurosis

loss of faith

despair

lack of self-respect

63

Using the Colour Violet

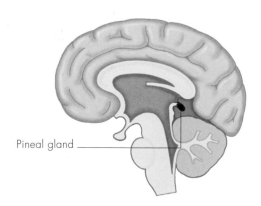

Pineal gland

Right brain
The colour violet is associated with the right side of the brain, the site of intuition, inner vision and clairvoyance.

Violet is the colour of the pineal gland, so-called because it is shaped like a pine cone. It is a pea-sized organ that is situated in the brain and it secretes melatonin and serotonin, the hormones that regulate our biological clock (see pages 24–25).

Violet vibrates at the highest frequency of all the colours of the spectrum and so it stimulates the highest expression of the human spirit. It is the colour of the mystic and, together with indigo, aids in the development of clairvoyance and psychic sensitivity.

Violet is a good colour for those of an artistic or highly strung temperament; such people tend to be naturally in tune with the colour's vibration. It also helps to soothe frayed nerves and bring peace to troubled minds. If you are feeling the strain of a modern, busy lifestyle, treatment with this colour can help to restore your sense of balance.

Masculine & feminine

Violet consists of both blue and red and, because of this, it helps to balance both ends of the colour spectrum. The warm colours are associated with the masculine energy and the cool with the feminine, so violet can help to bring these two energies into balance within a person.

The overall effect of violet is to unify body and mind with spirit, the demands of the mundane world with the need to feed the soul, and the inner with the outer. People who manage to achieve this unity know a peace that escapes many in our modern, materialistic society.

'Violet' people are also likely to know why they are here, and will have a sense of destiny, which often involves dedicating themselves in some way in the service of humanity. They make powerful and effective healers; if they are artists, their work speaks to the nature of the human condition in a way that all may understand.

However, violet has its negative expression and this takes the form of overweening pride and a sense of superiority. The power of this ray will backfire if it is not used wisely, in the service of others rather than to further your own ends.

Violet Qualities

Positive spiritual, noble, dignified, inspired, humble

Negative fanatical, perfectionist, self-doubting, self-destructive, alienated

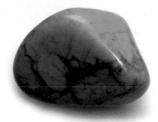

Turquoise
The turquoise stone contains copper and is a good conductor of healing.

TURQUOISE While not one of the seven rays, turquoise is an important healing colour. To many civilizations and peoples – the Atlanteans, Egyptians and Native Americans – both the colour and the stone were sacred and were worn for protection. Turquoise was thought to symbolize the heavens; the spirit as opposed to the flesh. Turquoise is a mix of blue and green, the colours of the sea, and it combines the qualities of both – the serenity of blue with the harmony of green.

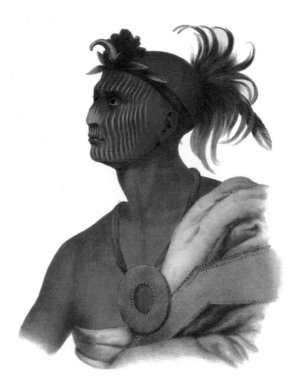

The sky
To Native Americans the colour turquoise symbolized the sky and the breath of life.

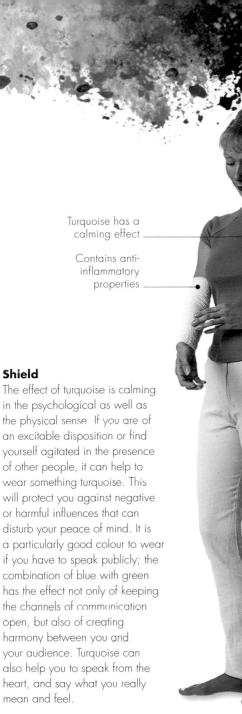

Turquoise has a calming effect

Contains anti-inflammatory properties

Healer

Like blue, turquoise has anti-inflammatory properties, and is a good colour to visualize (see pages 146–47) for a cut or burn because it helps to soothe and heal the wound. Turquoise is also known to help boost the immune system and it is a good colour to treat yourself with if you are suffering from a cold or the flu.

Shield

The effect of turquoise is calming in the psychological as well as the physical sense. If you are of an excitable disposition or find yourself agitated in the presence of other people, it can help to wear something turquoise. This will protect you against negative or harmful influences that can disturb your peace of mind. It is a particularly good colour to wear if you have to speak publicly; the combination of blue with green has the effect not only of keeping the channels of communication open, but also of creating harmony between you and your audience. Turquoise can also help you to speak from the heart, and say what you really mean and feel.

Turquoise Qualities

Positive composed, clear, creative, calm

Negative vain, boastful, confused

Turquoise Affirmation

'I express what I think and feel with clarity and conviction'.

Primary & Secondary Colours

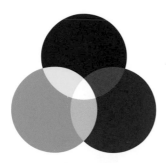

White light
If you project the colours red, green and blue on to the same spot, you will get white light.

Primary colours are so-called because all the other colours can be produced by using a mixture of them. However the definition of primary colours differs according to their source.

Colour in light

If the source is light, then the three primary colours are red, green and blue-violet, known as the additive colours, which, as Sir Isaac Newton discovered, combine to produce white light. If you direct three spotlights of these colours onto a white screen or wall, at the point where they overlap, you will see white light. When you combine two of these primary colours, you produce the secondary colours yellow, from red and green, cyan or turquoise from green and blue and magenta from red and blue-violet.

Colour in nature

So far only the colour of light has been discussed, but there is also pigment colour, which occurs, for instance, as chlorophyll in green plants and haemoglobin in red blood. Pigment has come to mean any substance that imparts colour and can be used to stain fabric, skin or hair, such as a dye.

There have always been natural dyes, such as indigo, woad and alizarin, which can be obtained from various plants, but the huge range of synthetic dyes available today dates from the middle of the last century.

Pigments & dyes

In the case of pigments or dyes, the primary colours are different to those of light. They are red, yellow and blue, and these are known as the subtractive colours.

If you mix the colours red, yellow and blue together, you produce black, because these colours absorb light. When you mix two of them together, you produce the secondary colours of orange (red mixed with yellow), green (yellow mixed with blue) and violet (red mixed with blue).

In addition to red, yellow and blue, the human eye also discerns green as a primary colour. If combined, these four colours produce a silver-grey.

The First Synthetic Dye

In 18.56, an Englishman, William Perkin, succeeded in making the first aniline dye from coal tar. This was mauve in colour and quickly led to the commercial production of hundreds of different coloured dyes.

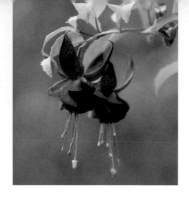

Fuchsia
*The vivid magenta flowers
of the fuchsia plant are
a voluptuous sight.*

MAGENTA This is a deep purplish red colour, made up of a combination of red and violet, and it is named after a town in Italy where a particularly bloody battle was fought in the mid-nineteenth century. It is also known as a brilliant crimson dye, sometimes referred to as fuchsin or fuchsine after the fuchsia flower. In modern times a bright magenta has been called a 'shocking' or a 'hot' pink.

A new start

If magenta starts appearing in your life, perhaps in the form of a new desire to wear the colour, you are now ready to let go of old habits or patterns in order to make way for the new. Magenta signifies change, the releasing of what we have outgrown in order to move on. Introducing magenta into your environment will help you to make changes, even if you just do something as simple as putting a fuchsia plant in your surroundings.

On the physical level magenta helps to energize the adrenal glands and the kidneys and it can also act as a diuretic. Its energy is calming and soothing and helps to stabilize people who are emotionally volatile or likely to be aggressive or violent.

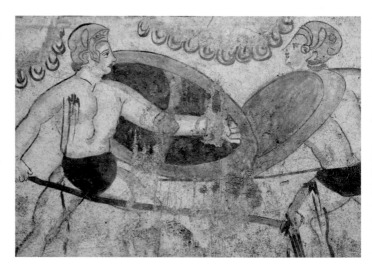

Battle
*The bright crimson of magenta is
the colour of blood shed in battle.*

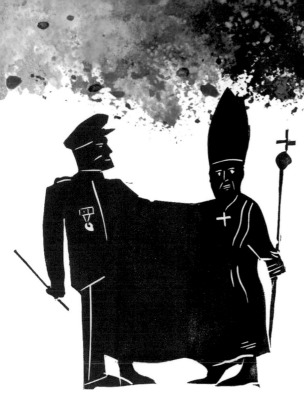

Strength & spirituality
The power of magenta derives from the strength of red and the spirituality of violet.

A transitional colour

Lying as it does between violet at one end of the colour spectrum and red at the other, magenta combines the qualities of both – the will and the authority of red with the spiritual power of violet. It is also the colour of transition, the place where we find ourselves between the ending of one cycle and the beginning of another.

Magenta Qualities

Positive open to change, mature, organized

Negative superior, self-righteous, insecure

Magenta Affirmation

'I have faith that everything will turn out for the best'.

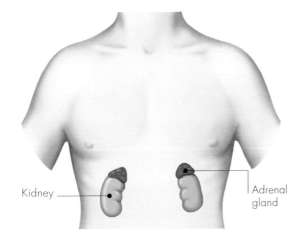

Kidney

Adrenal gland

Kidneys

The kidneys filter waste products from the blood, which are excreted as urine.

Tints & Shades

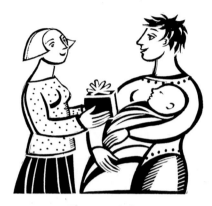

Blue & pink
It is traditional to give blue for a baby boy, and pink for a baby girl.

There are many subtle gradations of colour, which vary in tone from light to dark, bright to dull. Those with a proportion of white in them are called tints; those with a proportion of black, shades. Pale colours have more white in them, while dark colours contain more black.

We tend to wear paler colours in the summer, because they reflect the heat and are cooler, while darker colours are better in the winter because they absorb the heat and are warmer. The colours we wear also reflect our mood or convey the impression we want to make. We choose bright, vibrant colours for leisure, and sportswear, when we want to relax and have fun, while sombre colours are for more formal occasions, when we may have to keep our feelings in reserve.

Pink for a girl

All the colours of the spectrum have important tints and shades, with the exception of indigo, which does not have a tint. When we add white to red, for instance, we get pink, a soft and gentle colour associated with the feminine and unconditional love. Although we now dress children in a whole range of colours, it is still customary, when a little girl is born, to give her something pink.

Blue for a boy

Blue, at the other end of the spectrum, is for boys; the pale blue that mothers have traditionally dressed their little boys in is associated with the more spiritual and peace-loving aspects of the colour. The pastel colours of traditional babywear are protective, cocooning the child from too much stimulation too soon. Perhaps one of the reasons that children are growing up so quickly these days is that they are wearing much stronger and brighter colours at an earlier age than they used to.

Adding black to colour

When we add black to red, we get the darker, sludgy shades of red, associated with the more negative qualities of the colour, such as ruthlessness and brutality. Similarly, dark blue can denote a person who thinks he or she is always right, the dogmatist with set ideas. Generally speaking, the tints of a colour are positive, while the shades are more negative.

Colours in Tints & Shades

Tints are colours containing a proportion of white, such as peach, apricot, lemon, primrose, pink and light blue.

Shades are colours containing a proportion of black, such as dark blue and dark red.

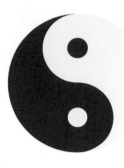

Balance
This ancient Eastern yin/ yang symbol represents balance between black and white, male and female.

BLACK is not, strictly speaking, a colour, because it absorbs light, but it is important because it is the opposite of white. Without darkness, there would be no light. However, there is in fact a pigment, melanin, from the Greek word *melas*, meaning black, which ranges from dark brown to black. This is present at a higher level in the hair, skin and eyes of black people and animals. Melanin is also responsible for tanning the skin and for melanomas, the tumours that occur when we overexpose our bodies to the sun.

Negative meanings
The word 'black' tends to have negative connotations, such as in the 'black sheep' of the family, the child who lets the other members down by behaving in a way that does not conform to their expectations. Then there are the 'black arts' or 'black magic', which involve invoking dark powers for evil ends. There is a seemingly endless list of terms with the word 'black' in them that have only bad meanings.

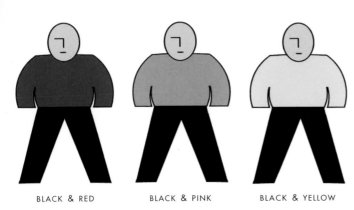

BLACK & RED   BLACK & PINK   BLACK & YELLOW

Positive

There is a positive side to black. It is considered lucky if a black cat crosses your path and to be 'in the black' with your bank account is better than being in the red. It is also one of the colours of the fertile earth and is associated with the Dark Moon, a very pregnant time. A seed planted then may grow to fruition at the Full Moon.

Black with other colours

Much of the superstition surrounding black is to do with its association with death, and also with power, which it lends to other colours when worn with them. Black with red denotes physical or sexual power; with pink, social status; and with yellow, mental superiority.

Black Qualities

Positive dramatic, dignified, discreet, powerful

Negative control freak, depressed, unapproachable

Black Affirmation

'I am in control of my life and no one can harm me'.

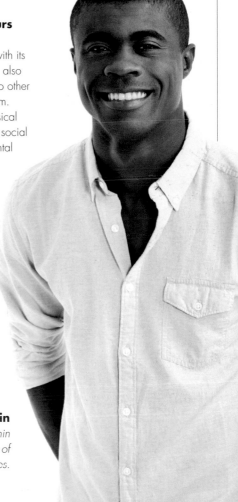

Melanin

The pigment melanin determines the colour of the skin, hair and eyes.

Wearing Black

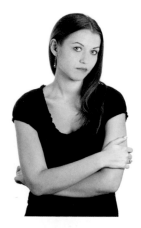

In control
Black clothes give the impression of being in control and remaining aloof from others.

Black has always had a place in the wardrobes of both men and women; it is the colour of mourning, of formal business suits and a favourite for glamorous evening wear. It has also become highly fashionable among the young, who dress in it from top to toe.

To wear black is to make a strong statement to others. When we don black for a funeral, we express sorrow for someone we have lost; when we wear a black suit to a business meeting, we tell our colleagues that we are in charge; and when we wear black in the evening, we say that we are alluring and mysterious.

Black confers dignity and power; the person who habitually wears black may seek to control others by keeping them at a distance, withholding information from them so that they do not gain either a psychological or a tactical advantage.

While the 'black' person may well stay 'on top', he or she may also have few close friends. Black has the effect of putting up a barrier between ourselves and other people, shutting them out and ultimately this can lead to feelings of isolation and even depression. To counter its negative effect, black should be worn with a splash of colour – perhaps by adding a tie, scarf, belt or shawl.

A protective colour

Black can also be protective and is a good colour to wear if you are feeling vulnerable and need to withdraw from the world for a while. Perhaps this is why it is such a popular colour with young people. The teenage boy or girl who will wear nothing but black is, after all, on the brink of a major threshold, from childhood to adulthood, which is one of the most difficult of transitions he or she has to make.

At this moment in history we are in the process of crossing over from one age to the next, which is the Age of Aquarius or the so-called New Age, with its increased emphasis on spirituality, holism and the environment. We are experiencing a high level of collective angst as we embark on a new millennium, not knowing what it will bring. This may well have something to do with the perennial popularity of black as a fashionable colour.

Goths

The epitome of worship of the colour black among the young was perhaps the 'Goth' fashion of the 1980s. This style was also echoed in the 2000s in the form of the 'Emo' fashion movement. Black velvet and leather featured strongly, together with jet black hair backcombed and hairsprayed into electric-shocked shapes to frame pancaked white skin and dramatic eye make-up. This was a look that was worn equally by boys and girls.

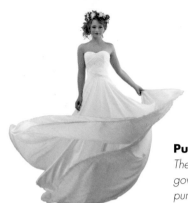

Purity
The white of the bridal gown symbolizes virginal purity and innocence.

WHITE
The pure white flowers of the snowdrop are a sign of hope on a dark winter day that spring is on its way. We tend to respond positively to white because it contains all the colours of the spectrum and reflects light. It is the colour of the bridal gown, a priest's vestments and the crests of the waves that are sometimes called white horses.

Positive meanings
In contrast to black, most common sayings with the word 'white' in them have positive meanings. A 'white lie' is usually told in order not to hurt someone's feelings and 'white magic', unlike black magic, is beneficent in purpose. To be 'whiter than white' is to be as pure as the driven snow, without a stain on your moral character.

White horses
We associate the white horses of a choppy sea with the tang of salt and a fresh wind.

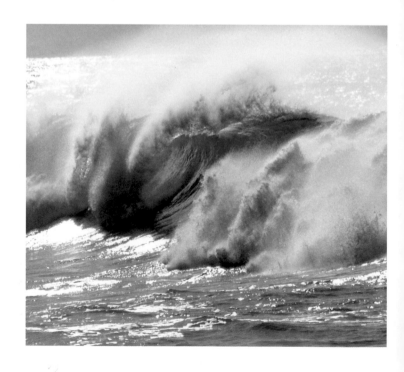

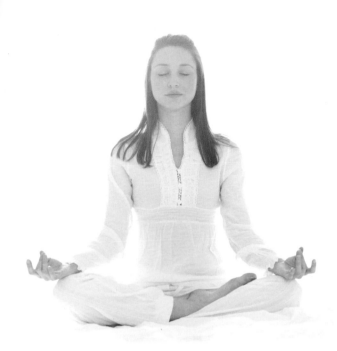

Spiritual

White is also associated with spirituality. Psychics and healers use white light to channel healing to those in need and you can meditate on it (see pages 140–43) to cleanse your system and give it a general boost. Many people who have come close to death as a result of illness or an accident in what are called near-death experiences, report being dazzled by white light.

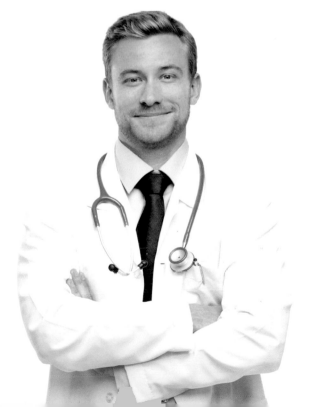

White Qualities

Positive pure, innocent, orderly, spiritual

Negative stark, critical, colourless

White Affirmation

'I have as much space as I need'.

The status of a white coat

Many health professionals wear white coats, and while in this context white conveys an impression of cleanliness, it can also suggest superiority. This can make others feel inadequate or ill at ease.

Living with White

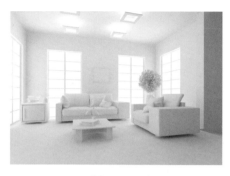

White room

A white living room may look light and spacious, but its starkness may not be conducive to relaxation.

White can be a difficult colour to live with. While a room decorated all in white may be striking in effect, it does not make the most comfortable of environments. White can be stark and unrelenting and needs to be offset by touches of colour in order for us to feel that we can relax.

Kitchens

A kitchen painted in white, for instance, may be light, cool and airy, but can also look very clinical; not the sort of room in which you feel like chatting over a cup of coffee with a friend. It needs to be balanced by coloured tiles or blinds, bowls of fruit and vegetables or jars of warm-hued spices and pulses.

Bathrooms

Similarly, a white bathroom can look and feel cold, not the kind of room where you want to take off your clothes, let alone soak in a long, hot bath.

While white walls can reflect sunlight, many modern bathrooms are squeezed into small, windowless spaces and the monotony of the white needs to be offset by brightly coloured tiles or towels, or a plant that will thrive in the humid conditions of a bathroom.

Bedrooms

White is also a popular colour for bedrooms because it is clean and refreshing. An over-emphasis on the colour, however, especially if your tastes are traditional and you like lots of crisp, starched white bedlinen or lace, can lead to the opposite of the effect you are trying to achieve. Instead of a room where you can take sanctuary from the hustle and bustle of everyday life, you may find that you have created a space that makes you feel lonely or cut off.

Try painting your bedroom in one of the shades of white, or off-white, that are now widely available. For example, a hint of peach or apricot will bring warmth to the room, while a blush of pink will aid rest. Curtains and pictures in a contrasting colour can also help to soften the effect of white, which, on its own, can be harsh and even alienating. Or you can experiment with lighting (see box below), which can be coordinated with soft furnishings.

Lighting Tricks

The starkness of an all-white room can be minimized by clever use of lighting. Use lamps to add soft pools of light, and choose shades in colours that cast a warm glow, such as russet, terracotta, gold, burgundy, raspberry or candy pink. Look for lampshade materials that allow light through, rather than just funnelling it out of the top and bottom of the shade.

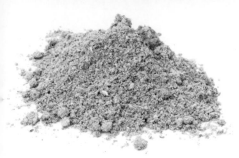

Ashes
*Grey ashes are all that is left
of the fire that has died.*

GREY is a combination of black and white but is neither one nor the other, hence its reputation for neutrality and even dullness. It is the colour of ashes and of lead as well as the hue of the sky on miserable days when it is raining and we don't know what to do with ourselves. At these times we may not be depressed, but we are not exactly buoyant either.

Negative meanings
A 'grey cloud on the horizon' indicates that something is on the way that may cast a shadow over the present. It is often something that we may fear, because we do not know what its outcome will be. A 'grey area' is something that we are uncertain about and we may therefore take a non-committal stance on it.

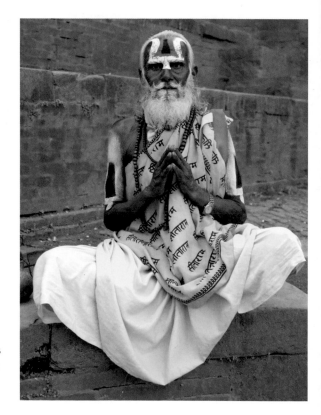

Positive meanings
Lying as it does between two extremes, grey has positive as well as negative meanings. It is the colour of intelligence, as in 'grey matter' or brain tissue. 'Greybeard' not only means old man, but often wise old man or sage, too.

Silvery grey

In silver, grey takes on an almost magical connotation; silver is the colour we associate with the moon and the feminine. It is used to describe films, as in 'silver screen' – here, we cannot be sure of anything we see, what is real and what is illusion – we are in the realm of the imagination and may therefore create our own reality.

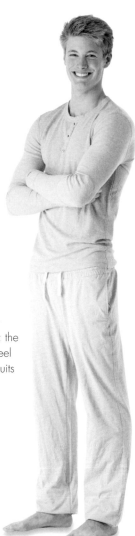

Leisure wear

Grey is also a popular colour for leisure wear; the clothes we relax and feel comfortable in – tracksuits and sweatshirts – are often made in various shades of grey.

Grey Qualities

Positive safe, impartial, restful, wise

Negative uninteresting, indecisive, dismal

Grey Affirmation

'I take the time to make up my mind about where I want to go'.

Tint & Shade Secrets

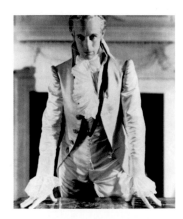

Scarlet Pimpernel
The colour scarlet is bright and bold, the colour of he who dares, despite the consequences.

Generally speaking, the clear, bright, strong hues of a colour signify its most positive qualities, while the darker shades denote its more negative attributes. The pastel tints tend to stand for the colour at its highest expression.

Red

We have already looked at pink as a tint of red as well as the darker shades of red; in between are the vivid crimson and scarlet. Crimson stands for strength and tenacity, while scarlet is associated with boldness and courage. An example of the latter is the Scarlet Pimpernel, the English nobleman who smuggled aristocrats out of France during the French Revolution. However, the colour is also associated with lust and sexual promiscuity, as summed up in the expression 'scarlet woman'.

Orange & yellow

Peach and apricot, being tints of orange, are both positive in meaning. They are warm colours that induce a sense of well-being so are good to wear if you have to communicate with people or need their cooperation. Darker shades of orange indicate self-gratification or underachievement.

The pale yellows, lemon and primrose, bring out the best qualities of yellow – a good mind, discerning judgment and the ability to distinguish truth from falsehood. This is the colour of the intellectual, the philosopher, the person who searches for meaning. Dark yellow, on the other hand, is associated with a suspicious mind, destructive criticism and malice. This is the colour of the person who likes to pick a fight or who may be vindictive.

Green

Bright emerald green is one of the
most positive colours in the spectrum,
suggesting an abundance of what we
need and generosity with what we have.
It is associated with giving and receiving
freely, so that all may be in balance. Pale
greens relate to qualities of the heart, like
sympathy, kindness and compassion.
Again, these are given without thought
of what might be gained in return. Dark
greens, however, are indicative of the
darker emotions – envy, bitterness and
possessiveness.

The Message of Tints

This checklist shows the key characteristics of
these tints.

scarlet lust

peach good communication

lemon clear mind

emerald abundance

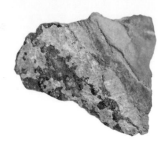

Tiger's eye
*The brown and yellow
of tiger's eye are the
colours of the Earth.*

BROWN This colour has a plethora of associations with the Earth – everything from soil to rocks and minerals, the bark of trees, autumn leaves, seeds and nuts. In the human and animal world, too, it features strongly – it is a dominant colour of skin, hair and eyes. The tiger's-eye stone, with its rich coppery colours, has many of the qualities that we associate with brown. It has a steadying influence, which helps us to stay on the straight and narrow; it also helps us to concentrate our energies on the task in hand, rather than dissipating them in all directions.

Nostalgia
Perhaps because of its
association with autumn,
brown can be associated with
melancholy and nostalgia, but
these are natural feelings, which
need to be valued for what they
are. We cannot be bright and
happy all the time, any more than
we can have eternal spring.

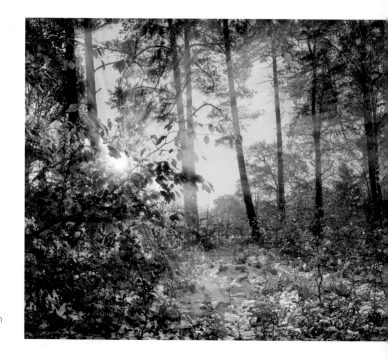

Mother Earth

Brown is the colour of Mother Earth, which nourishes and sustains us all in a never-ending cycle of birth and death, growth and decay. In spring we plant seed, in summer we harvest fruit and in autumn the leaves on the trees wither to brown and fall to become mulch for the next cycle. At this time of year we might wander through the woods in a 'brown study' or reverie, absorbed in our own thoughts.

Reliable

We tend to take brown for granted, because it is always there, like the furniture of our homes, solid and reassuring. But without it our lives would lack stability. It is one of the colours favoured in business, because of its association with reliability and a practical, common-sense approach. Most of us have worn the colour at one time or another, even if only in the form of a pair of shoes, or an accessory like a handbag or watchstrap.

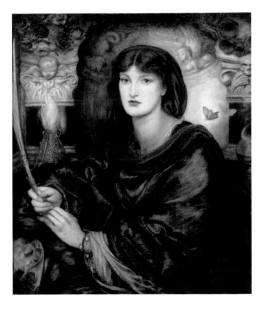

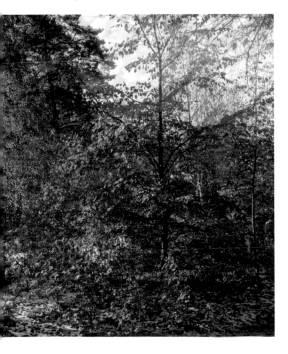

Grounding

Brown is a good colour to wear if you are feeling unfocused and need to ground yourself; or if you feel at the mercy of outside influences and need to protect yourself. However wearing too much of this colour can make you afraid to embrace change and anything new or unfamiliar.

Brown Qualities

Positive secure, enduring, stable, industrious

Negative conservative, fearful, boring

Brown Affirmation

'I am secure in myself and have everything that I need'.

Tint & Shade Wisdom

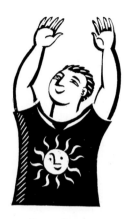

Devotion
*Blue is the colour of devotion, whether
to God, art or a worthy cause.*

On pages 72–73 and 84–85 we examined the meanings given to some tints and shades. Now we take a look at the meanings of blue, indigo and violet.

Blue

Pale blue is traditionally associated with baby boys; however, this particular blue is also blue at its most ethereal and it represents devotion to a high ideal. Deep blue, on the other hand, symbolizes the best of 'blue' qualities: loyalty, integrity and trustworthiness.

The darker shades of blue, like those of most colours, carry a negative connotation, with the exception of navy blue, which is so-called because of its association with naval uniforms. This colour stands for authority and sober judgment, which may be one of the reasons it is so often chosen for formal business clothing.

Indigo has no tint, but black mixed with this colour can, for instance, turn an inspired teacher into a cult leader who demands blind obedience from his or her followers. Similarly, a deep, dark purple is associated with the high-ranking official who has been corrupted by power and abuses the position of their office.

The lighter purples like lavender, lilac and amethyst bring out blue's more mystical, healing and aesthetic properties, symbolizing the highest expression of which we are capable.

The hidden meaning of colour

All colours, with the exception of the primary colours, are a made up of a mixture of other colours. Orange is made up of red and yellow, yellow consists of red and green, green is a combination of blue and yellow and so on. It is important, when using colours for healing purposes, to be aware of the colours that go to make up a particular colour, because the body will experience the vibrations coming from all these colours.

So if you are treating yourself with the colour green, for example, you will not only experience the harmony of green itself, but also the calming influence of blue and the mental stimulation of yellow. This is what makes green such a good colour for healing, because it balances both ends of the colour spectrum.

Sensing Colour

The primary way that we sense colour is obviously through the eyes; however, we also sense it subconsciously through the skin.

It is possible to develop this sensitivity in order to identify colours by touching them with our hands. Indeed, many blind people are able to differentiate colours in this way.

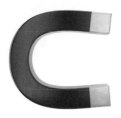

Opposites attract
Opposites attract, whether the poles of a magnet or complementary colours.

COMPLEMENTARY COLOURS
Each colour has its complementary colour, which lies opposite to it on the colour wheel (see page 35). While green is the complementary colour to red, for healing purposes it is blue that is used. A colour and its complementary colour balance and attract each other like poles of a magnet, which is a very important consideration in colour healing.

'Seeing' the complementary colour

Even without looking at the colour wheel, you can see the complementary colours for yourself by doing a very simple exercise. Stare hard at a red object, for instance, for a few seconds and then look away to a sheet of white paper or a white wall. You will see the after-image appear on the white in the form of the complementary colour, in this case green. This has its counterpoint in nature, in the second rainbow we can sometimes see in the sky. It appears above the first rainbow, but if you look closely at it, you will see that its colours are in reverse order, with the blue colours at the bottom of the arc and the red at the top.

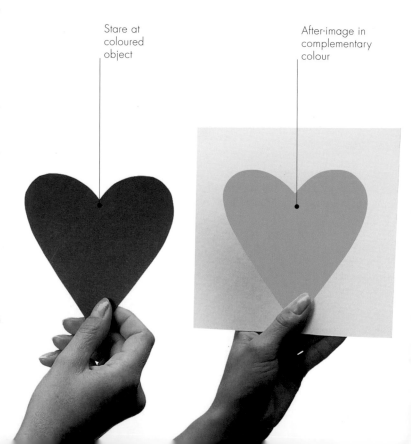

Stare at coloured object

After-image in complementary colour

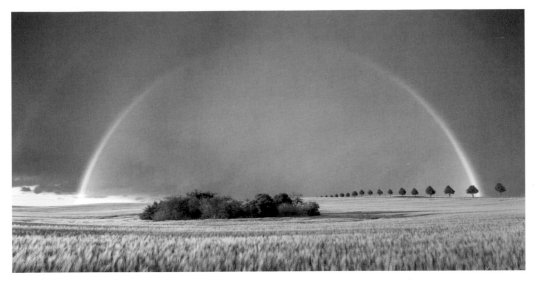

Rainbow

To see how the colours complement one another, you have only to look at the rainbow that appears in the sky after a storm, arcing over the land in a vivid display of colour.

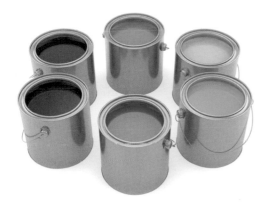

Complementary Colours			
red	green	blue	red
orange	indigo	indigo	orange
yellow	violet	violet	yellow

Mixed colours

It is a little harder to see the complementary colours in colours that have been mixed, such as with paint. If you are looking around a room at home and feel that the colours are out of balance, but are not sure what other colours to introduce, you can carry out the same simple test described opposite. Just stare at the wall or the sofa in the colour that is disturbing you and then look away to a sheet of white paper. You will see its complementary colour and this is what you need to match as nearly as possible in some way in the room, in order to coordinate your colour scheme.

Generally speaking, the lighter the tint, the darker the shade that is required to complement it.

Complementary Colours in Healing

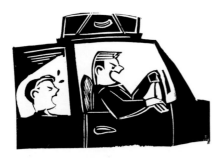

Stress

If you find yourself in a stressful situation, the colour blue will help you keep your temper.

Any disease or disharmony within the body shows up as an imbalance of colour energy. For example, if you are suffering from high blood pressure or are feeling angry or irritable, then there is an excess of red energy in your system. The appropriate colour to treat yourself with is the complementary colour, blue.

It may be that you are sitting in a traffic jam, fuming at the delay as you need to keep an important appointment. You obviously will not have access to coloured lamps or filters but you can meditate on blue (see pages 140–43), or even just look out of the window at the blue sky. You will find that your anger dissipates and you begin to calm down.

Likewise, you may go to a beauty salon for a relaxing massage and find that the treatment room is decorated in yellow. As even the pale tones of this colour can be over-stimulating, ask the therapist if he or she has a purple towel that can be put over you or, while you are lying there, visualize the colour purple (see pages 146–47). You will soon find that the decor ceases to disturb you.

Treatment times

This principle of treatment with complementary colours is all-important in colour healing and also extends to ensuring you treat the complementary colour with its own complementary colour at the end of a colour healing session. For example, if you are receiving treatment with blue for, say, high blood pressure or stress – which are red conditions – then it will be necessary to have treatment with red in order to complete the session.

Many colour therapists, particularly those
using lamps or filters in their treatment, have
exposure times to all the different colours
worked out to the minute, or fraction of a
minute. It is wise, if you are considering
doing a treatment for yourself, to consult
a qualified colour healer first about how
long to treat yourself with each colour.

Green

If you are ever in doubt about the effects
of a colour, or feel you have exposed
yourself for too long to a particular colour,
you can always treat yourself with green,
or even just visualize it, to remedy the
situation. Green, being a neutral colour,
will correct any imbalance you have
inadvertently created.

METHODS OF COLOUR HEALING

In this section of the book you will be introduced to methods of colour healing that you can try out for yourself without going to any great expense or trouble. It may be that you are feeling dispirited or stressed, or are suffering from some kind of physical illness. Whatever it is, you are likely to be aware of an imbalance of energy within yourself that treatment by colour can heal. Some of the methods that are described go back to ancient times, like colour breathing or drinking coloured water; others are more modern, involving the use of lamps or coloured filters. However they are all relatively simple and easy to practise. Remember that colour healing by itself is not necessarily going to put matters right and, if you have a serious health problem, it is important that you consult your doctor or another qualified health professional.

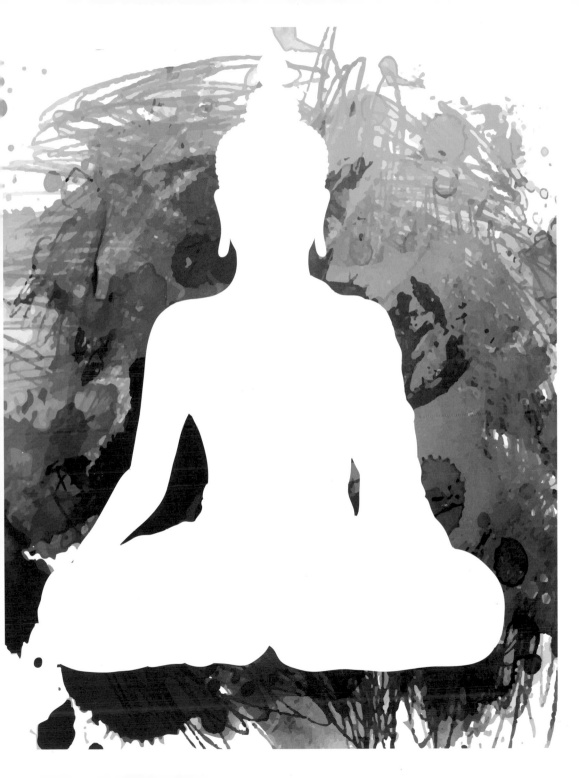

The Aura

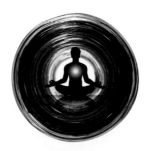

Bands of colour
The human body is surrounded by light or energy in bands of different colours, known as the aura.

An aura is the light or energy that emanates from the body of a human being or animal; it is also thought to be emitted by plants, stones and any visible object.

An aura is usually described as being shaped like an egg, or an oval, and, in most people, it extends 5–8 centimetres (2–3 inches) around the body in different layers or bands, in different colours. The band nearest the body is called the etheric sheath, also known as the etheric double, because it is the counterpart of the physical body. The etheric sheath draws vital life force from the atmosphere and distributes it through the chakras or energy centres (see pages 100–101) in the body.

Reading the aura

The aura says a great deal about a person's physical, mental and emotional state, and spiritual development. The size and condition of the aura varies – the more highly evolved someone is, the larger and more radiant their aura is likely to be. Conversely, the aura of a person who is not well or whose energy levels are low, may appear duller and smaller than normal.

In the early twentieth century, Dr W. J. Kilner invented a device that came to be known as the Kilner screen. This was a kind of lens, consisting of two pieces of glass, between which a solution of an indigo-violet dye was poured, enabling Kilner and his colleagues allegedly to perceive the aura of their patients and to make their diagnosis accordingly. An excess of red might indicate stress, for example, for which treatment with blue was appropriate; an abundance of blue meant a lack of energy, for which treatment with red was appropriate.

Kirlian photography

In 1939 a Russian scientist, Semyon Kirlian, claimed to have discovered a way of photographing the energy field of humans and other living things, by applying a high voltage current to an object on a photographic plate. This aroused interest in the aura as a means of diagnosis. Kirlian demonstrated that a photograph taken of a leaf just after it was picked, showed a bright, clear energy field, but one taken an hour later showed the field had diminished in size and colour. But the reasons for this are disputed by scientists and, as a diagnostic tool Kirlian photography remains controversial.

The Weather Vane of the Soul

The famous American clairvoyant, Edgar Cayce, put it beautifully when he said that for him, 'the aura is the weather vane of the soul. It shows which way the winds of destiny are blowing'.

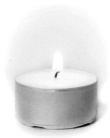

Shimmer
The aura of a candle is the faint shimmer around it.

HOW TO SEE AN AURA
Nowadays you can walk into a mind, body and spirit festival, sit down in front of a computer and have your aura photographed in seconds. However it is possible, with a little practice, even if you are not a natural psychic or sensitive, to train yourself to see the auras of other people with your own eyes.

Focusing on an aura

Most of us are familiar with the experience of looking at a lighted candle and after a few moments, seeing a faint, fuzzy shimmer all around it. This is the aura or corona of the candle. Part of being able to see auras is the ability to keep looking at something while remaining relaxed. The meditation techniques described on pages 140–45 will help you to do this. You can try this with someone you know. Focus on some part of their upper body, such as their mouth or their ears and then let your gaze relax. After a while you may begin to see a glow around their head and shoulders, and then their whole body. Eventually you may be able to see different colours emanating from different parts of their body.

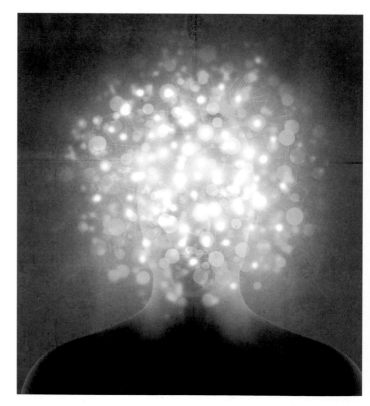

The clues to health

Aura colours will vary according to the person's general state of health and how they are feeling at the time, but you will soon learn to interpret them. In the aura of someone who is ill or depressed, for instance, the colours are likely to be very dark or subdued; in the aura of someone who is angry, there is likely to be a lot of red; and in the aura of someone who is a healer or a counsellor, for example, you may well see purple, which is the colour of service to others.

Aura vision

With practice, you may be able to develop the ability to see auras. Try this with a friend.

Dark-green aura
This person may be feeling bitter, envious or resentful.

Meditation brings benefits

Learn to be receptive

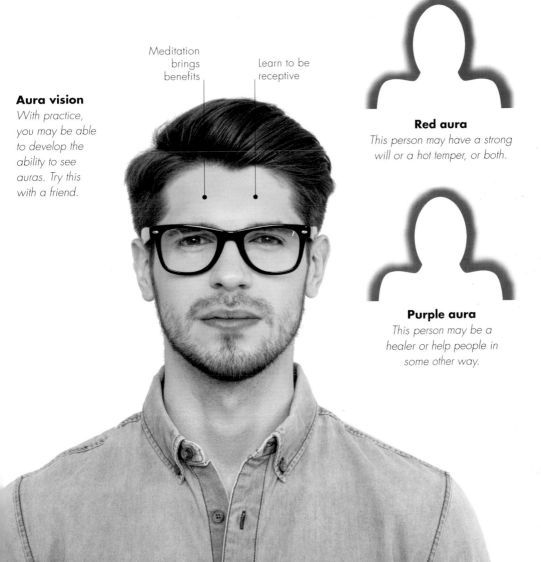

Red aura
This person may have a strong will or a hot temper, or both.

Purple aura
This person may be a healer or help people in some other way.

The Chakras

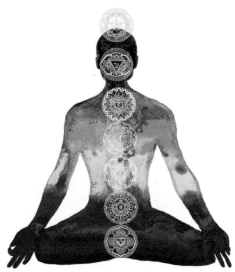

The major chakras

Five of the major chakras are aligned with the spine and they all relate to specific energies.

The different bands of the aura relate to the seven main chakras. 'Chakra' is a Sanskrit word, meaning 'wheel' and these energy centres spin clockwise or anticlockwise, according to whether they are absorbing energy or releasing it.

Each chakra is located in a particular part of the body and is associated with a corresponding organ or gland. They are also related to particular properties: physical, emotional and spiritual.

The seven energy centres

The root or base chakra is located at the base of the spine and is associated with the lower part of the body – the legs, feet and intestines. It is also related to the reproductive organs. Our sense of reality, ability to fend for ourselves in the world and overall vitality depend on this chakra.

The sacral chakra is located in the pelvic area, just below the navel, and is the body's sexual energy centre. It is associated with the liver, pancreas, spleen, kidneys and bladder, and as such, regulates bodily fluids. It is related to how well we feel.

Above the navel is the solar plexus chakra, which is associated with the stomach and the functioning of the sympathetic nervous system (this speeds up nerve responses). This chakra governs the passions, or 'gut feelings' and it also influences our sense of personal power.

The heart chakra is situated in the centre of the chest and relates to the thymus gland, which plays a vital role in the immune system. It regulates our emotional balance and rules love, compassion and kindness.

The throat chakra is at the front of the throat and is connected to the thyroid gland, which controls the body's metabolism. It is the centre of speech, communication and self-expression.

The brow chakra, between the eyebrows in the centre of the forehead, is associated with the pituitary gland, which controls the body's hormone production. This chakra is known as the third eye, because it sees clairvoyantly.

The crown chakra is on the top of the head. This is connected to the pineal gland, which influences the unconscious processes. The crown chakra is the centre of spirituality or the soul.

Nadis

The chakras are linked by nadis, from another Sanskrit word, meaning 'hollow stalk'. Nadis are energy channels through which the prana, the breath of life, flows around the body. There are numerous nadis in the body, and they correspond to the acupuncture meridians.

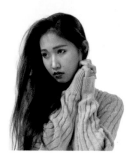

Blocked energy
If someone is ill or feeling negative, the chakra colours will be weaker and dimmer, and energy flow blocked. Disharmony will show in the aura.

COLOURS OF THE CHAKRAS
The etheric sheath, which surrounds the physical body, acts rather like a prism, refracting light into the colours of the spectrum, that then resonate with the chakras. The colour of the base chakra is red; of the sacral chakra, orange; of the solar plexus chakra, yellow; of the heart chakra, green; of the throat chakra, blue; of the brow chakra, indigo; and of the crown chakra, violet.

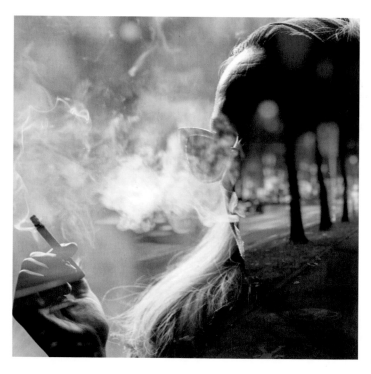

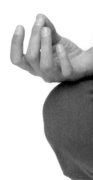

Aura damage
The aura of a smoker or alcoholic will contain little specks of 'dust', showing pollution to the system.

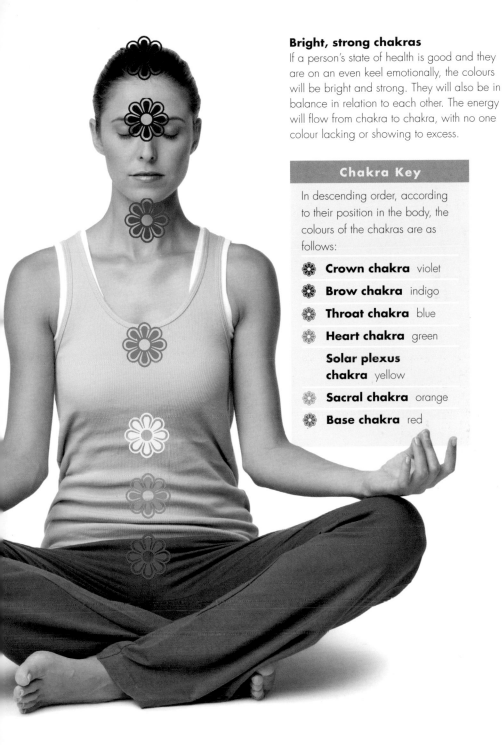

Bright, strong chakras

If a person's state of health is good and they are on an even keel emotionally, the colours will be bright and strong. They will also be in balance in relation to each other. The energy will flow from chakra to chakra, with no one colour lacking or showing to excess.

Chakra Key

In descending order, according to their position in the body, the colours of the chakras are as follows:

- **Crown chakra** violet
- **Brow chakra** indigo
- **Throat chakra** blue
- **Heart chakra** green
- **Solar plexus chakra** yellow
- **Sacral chakra** orange
- **Base chakra** red

Blockages in the Chakras

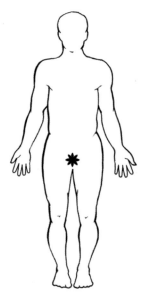

Base chakra

A blockage in the base chakra impairs the vital life force leading to feelings of exhaustion.

cannot accept or let go of, will have grey in them; this might even actually show up as a knot or ball. In this context, grey is the colour of fear and doubt; however, it is also the colour of transition and indicates the possibility of change.

If the base chakra is affected, we may find that we lack the energy to do things, or we may suffer from chronic lower back pain. These physical problems, in turn, may be related to feelings of insecurity or being unsupported in the world. An excess of energy in this area could lead to violent, uncontrolled behaviour.

If the sacral chakra is not functioning properly, both sexes may experience a variety of problems in the pelvic region, or may experience problems in sexual relationships.

Blockages in the solar plexus chakra may show up physically as ulcers or other stomach problems, indigestion, diabetes or hepatitis. The psychological problems that may occur include stress or anxiety. Because the solar plexus chakra is related to our mentality, there may also be difficulty in thinking clearly or taking decisions.

When our feelings are blocked and the flow of energy is restricted through the chakras, we do not function well either physically or psychologically. This manifests in different ways according to the chakra that is affected. The auras of people who are blocked in an emotional or psychological sense, perhaps as a result of feelings they

Higher chakra problems

Any disturbance in the action of the heart
chakra is likely to result in heart or lung
problems. It may also cause difficulties
in relationships, because a problem here
inhibits the expression of love. This in turn
may be related to a lack of self-love as
well as a mistrust of other people.

Blockages in the throat chakra tend to
manifest as thyroid problems, laryngitis or
a sore throat. They can also cause difficulty
in voicing things or speaking up for
ourselves, or we may be very opinionated
and insist that others share our views.

If the brow chakra is unstable, we may
suffer from insomnia, fatigue, headaches
or nervous disorders. We may also not
trust our intuition or capacity to perceive
other realities.

Dysfunction of the crown chakra is
also associated with nervous disorders,
including multiple sclerosis. It is also related
to a lack of spiritual awareness and a
feeling that life has little or no meaning.

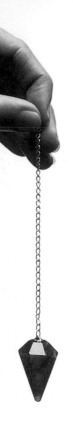

Answer
Using a pendulum can help you find your own answer to a question.

DOWSING
If you feel that something is not quite right, either physically or emotionally, but are not sure what colour you need to help rebalance your energies, then you can always try dowsing to find out which one you should use. To do this, you will need a pendulum, which you can easily make yourself.

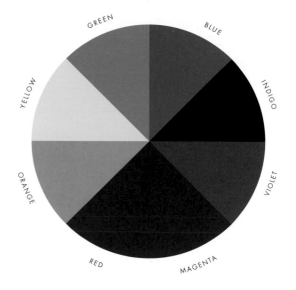

Making & using a pendulum
To create a pendulum use a crystal that you feel particularly drawn to. Tie a piece of string or cord around it, making sure that there is enough slack to be able to dangle it. Then, unless you want to make your own colour wheel, turn to the colour wheel on page 35 as you will need it later.

Now you need to find out how the pendulum will work for you. Ask, out loud or in your mind, which way it is going to swing for a 'yes' answer. After a second or two, the pendulum will begin to move, in a clockwise or anticlockwise direction, or from side to side. Do the same for a 'no', and perhaps also for a 'don't know, try again' answer.

Colour wheel
This colour wheel includes magenta, which lies between red and violet.

Colour dowsing

Now you are ready to dowse for the colour you need. First of all, be clear about the question you want to ask and frame it in such a way that the answer has to be a yes or a no. For example, you might be feeling a bit low, but not sure which of the warm colours you need. You could simply ask, 'Do I need red/orange/yellow?' Then hold the pendulum over the colour wheel and see in which direction it swings. It may be that it actually goes to the colour you need. Then all you have to do is choose one of the methods of colour healing described in the rest of this section.

Ask the question
in your mind

Intuition

The beauty of this method is that you are using your own intuition and not relying on an expert or somebody else for the answer.

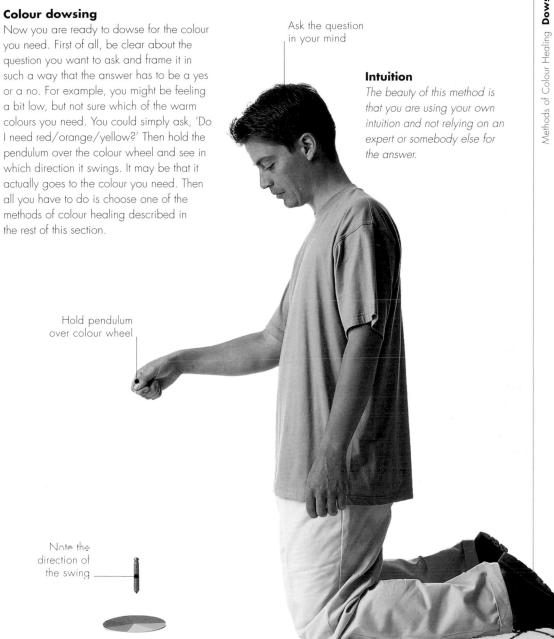

Hold pendulum
over colour wheel

Note the
direction of
the swing

Healing with Coloured Light

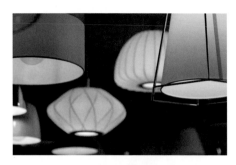

Atmosphere
Coloured light is a very effective way of creating the atmosphere that you want in any room in the home.

Coloured light healing is also known as chromatherapy, from the Greek word *khroma*, meaning light. This form of healing goes back to ancient times and the use of glass or crystals to filter the rays of the sun. Nowadays you can buy a variety of lamps for specific healing purposes. There is a lamp that will illuminate your surroundings with the colour you require, whether it is blue for relaxation or orange for socializing, and so on.

However, without spending a lot of money, you can also create your own coloured lamp by buying coloured filters or gels from a specialist lighting or photography supplier. These can then be placed over an ordinary lamp at home, although care should be taken to leave a gap between the filter and the bulb, otherwise the filter will burn.

Alternatively you can buy coloured light bulbs, which are widely available, and fit them to lamps that you already have. If your bedroom is a cold room, for example, fit an apricot- or peach-coloured bulb in your bedside lamp, for a warm glow that will suffuse the room.

Candlelight
Another cheap but effective method is to burn a candle or tea light in a coloured glass. If you are feeling stressed or harassed, for example, try placing a candle in a blue or indigo-coloured glass; it will calm you down and it is also particularly good for meditation. Candlelight is soft and gentle and, when combined with coloured glass, can help to induce a particular mood or feeling.

Treatment
Treatment with coloured light usually takes two forms: it can be diffused over the whole body, especially the back, and this is generally used as a revitalizer; or it can

be concentrated on one particular spot,
where you feel out of balance or there is
disease. If you are not sure what colour
to treat yourself with, try dowsing for it,
or refer to the previous section of this book
for lists of specific conditions and states
of mind that are helped by treatment
with a particular colour.

The Nature of Light

Light travels through space in waves, at different
frequencies according to the colour. Violet
radiates in short waves and pacifies, while red
radiates in long waves and invigorates.

USING COLOURED LIGHT
If you want to treat a specific part of your body with coloured light, it is probably best to go to a trained colour therapist, who will be able to ascertain what colour you need and, most importantly, how long you should be exposed to it. Generally speaking, white or very light clothing should be worn during treatment, because this helps you to absorb the colour better. If you wear a particular colour, it may interfere with the treatment.

Light sources
There are specially manufactured light instruments, which are safe to use so long as you follow the instructions carefully. If, however, you just want to create a general effect of healing, then you can put a coloured filter over a lamp or a coloured light bulb in it, whether its a free-standing lamp, a bedside lamp or an angle-poise lamp.

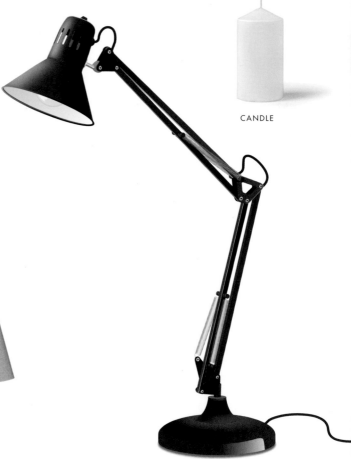

CANDLE

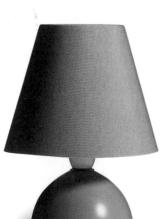

BEDSIDE LAMP

ANGLE-POISE LAMP

Light treatment

It can be dangerous to expose yourself to colour for too long, particularly if it is at the red or hot end of the spectrum, otherwise you may end up creating an imbalance in your body. The treatment also needs to be completed with exposure to the complementary colour for a shorter period. As a general rule, treatment with green and colours at the blue end of the spectrum should not exceed 15 minutes, while treatment with red should only be for less than half that time. Treatment with the complementary colour varies between 3 minutes for red and blue and 7 for green and magenta.

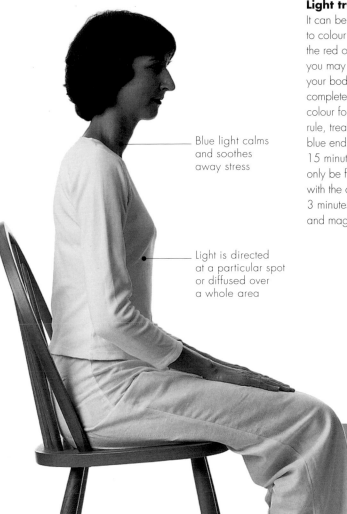

Blue light calms and soothes away stress

Light is directed at a particular spot or diffused over a whole area

Exposure Time

If you are in any doubt about the time for which you should expose yourself to a particular colour, a qualified colour therapist will be able to help, particularly if you have a condition that would benefit from regular treatments.

Healing with Coloured Water

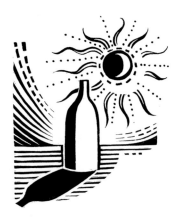

Sun's rays
*Water is energized by exposing
a coloured bottle filled with water
to the rays of the sun.*

This is one of the oldest methods of colour healing and it is still practised today in India by doctors of Ayurvedic medicine, as a way of introducing colour into the body to alleviate its aches and pains. Quite simply, this method involves filling a coloured container of some kind with water and placing it in the path of the sun, a process that is known as solarization. The sun's rays will then energize the water with the qualities of the colour you have chosen. The ancient Egyptians made exquisite pottery jars of blue faience for this purpose.

The modern equivalent of the Egyptian jar can be seen today in the bottles and jars, made out of glass or plastic, that are used to package water, fruit juice and various other soft drinks. A lot of mineral or spring water, for instance, is sold in bottles of varying hues of blue and green. These colours are deliberately chosen by the manufacturers for their cooling and thirst-quenching properties: try drinking water from a clear glass or bottle and then from a blue or green glass or bottle. Many people find that water from the latter tastes colder and fresher.

Decanting other liquids

This principle applies to other liquids besides water. You can decant milk, medicine, oil, lotion and so on into a container of the appropriate colour to enhance its effect. You might, for example, pour milk into an orange glass for a tonic drink first thing in the morning; cough mixture into a green bottle to help relieve the symptoms of colds or flu; or lavender body lotion into a purple container to augment its soothing and relaxing properties. You can even apply this principle to storing beans, pulses or other foodstuffs in appropriately coloured jars.

Generally speaking, drinking water that has been solarized with the red ray has an energizing or warming effect; while the orange ray has a vitalizing effect; the yellow ray, a stimulating effect; the green ray, a balancing or stabilizing effect; and blue, indigo or violet rays, a soothing effect.

The Sun God Ra

The priests of ancient Egypt placed bowls of fruit and vegetable juice in the sun to absorb the energy of the sun god, Ra. The bowls were also set with jewels of the same colour as the fruit and vegetables to enhance the effect.

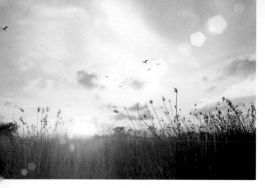

Sunrise
The sun rises on another day, bringing light, energy and heat.

USING COLOURED WATER
Drinking solarized water is one of the safest ways to absorb colour into the system. Once you have decided on the colour you need, all you have to do is to fill a glass, jug or other container with water and expose it to direct sunlight through a filter of the relevant colour. Leave it to absorb the light for at least an hour. The water will retain its efficacy for a couple of days if you keep it refrigerated. Use a bottle or jar with a screw-top lid.

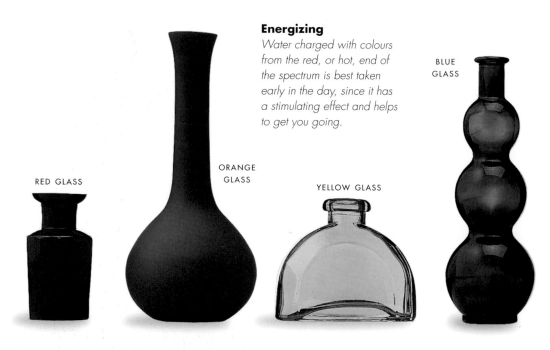

Energizing
Water charged with colours from the red, or hot, end of the spectrum is best taken early in the day, since it has a stimulating effect and helps to get you going.

BLUE GLASS

RED GLASS

ORANGE GLASS

YELLOW GLASS

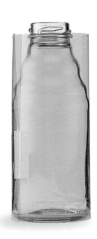

Making solarized water

To make solarized water it is best to use mineral water, or water that has been passed through a water filter. You can tape or clip the coloured filter around the glass or, alternatively, use a coloured glass or bottle. Then put it out in the sun, perhaps on a windowsill, to absorb the light through the colour, so that the water becomes charged with it. You will need to let the glass or bottle stand for up to an hour in direct sunlight, and even longer if it is not a sunny day. The water will keep fresh in the fridge for two to three days and can then be taken as required.

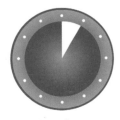

One hour
One hour in the sun should be long enough to solarize water.

Taste

You will find that water that has been solarized with one of the colours from the blue end of the spectrum tastes different from water solarized with one of the colours from the red end of the spectrum, and stays fresher longer.

Calming

Green, blue, indigo and violet solarized water is best taken later in the day, since it has a calming effect.

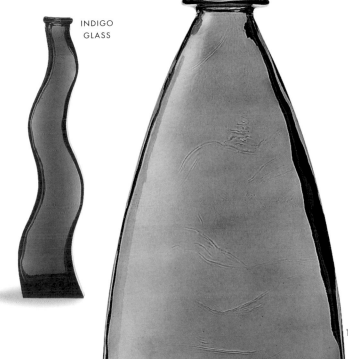

VIOLET GLASS

INDIGO GLASS

GREEN GLASS

Colour Baths

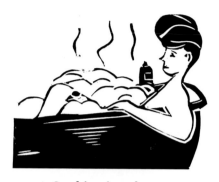

Soaking in colour
*Soaking in a colour bath is a
particularly pleasant and relaxing
form of colour healing.*

Another way of absorbing the energy
of colour is to take a colour bath.
This can take different forms –
you can use dyes or food colourings to
turn the water the colour that you want. If
you do not like the idea of this, you can
add bath salts, flowers, flower essences,
herbs or essential oils to the water.

There are many different kinds of foam
baths and bath gels, but most of these are
synthetic and are sold for their scent alone.
Some products contain essential oils, which
are very beneficial because they are
100 per cent natural. They are not only
absorbed through the skin, but the scent
can be inhaled from the warm bath water.

If you add essential oils to a colour bath
yourself, remember that only a very few
drops are needed. Read the instructions
on the bottle and follow them carefully.

Fragrance with colour

Oils can also be added to salts for
different combinations to relieve stress,
clear the mind or just to help you to feel
good about yourself. The combination
of fragrance with colour is especially
healing, so if you find yourself drawn to a
particular flower for its scent and the effect
it has on you, you might wish to throw a
few of its petals into your bath as well.
Try throwing in a handful or two of pink
rose petals to give you a sense of well-
being. Or float some stems of freesia on
the water; their heavenly scent gives rise
to an uplifting feeling. Freesias come in
many different colours, so you can choose
the colour according to the feeling that
you want to induce.

Flower essences

Flower essences are made from flowers
that have been energized by being
placed in pure water and exposed to
the direct light of the sun. They are

then combined with alcohol to make
a tincture. They are perhaps best
known as the products sold as the Bach
Flower Remedies. These are named
after Dr Edward Bach, the man whose
research between the years 1928 and
1932 gave us this form of healing.

Bach divided his remedies into
seven groups, each one associated with
a different colour, to alleviate various
negative states of mind. These remedies,
too, can be added to a colour bath for
the desired effect.

Edward Bach

Bach was working in the London Homeopathic
Hospital after the First World War, when he
observed that people's illnesses seemed to be
related to their personality. Negative moods
and attitudes appeared to have contributed to
their diseases. Bach set about developing the
remedies to address these negative states.

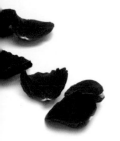

Flower petals

A few coloured flower petals in a bath can enhance the effect.

TAKING A COLOUR BATH When you take a colour bath, it is important not to run the water too hot, otherwise it interferes with the effect of the colour energy you are using and, if you are adding an essential oil, could also cause that to evaporate. You can have the water temperature a bit higher for a red, orange or yellow bath, but it should be lower for a green, blue, indigo or violet bath. It is, in any case, not a good idea to run too hot a bath because it is bad for the heart. A moderate temperature, close to body temperature, is best.

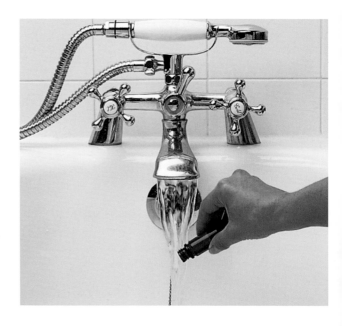

Essential oils

If you are adding an essential oil to your bath, sprinkle a few drops of it over the water once you have run it; if you are adding bath salts, throw them in and make sure that they have dissolved before you step into the water. Then soak in the bath for a while, at least 10 or 15 minutes, to allow yourself to absorb the energy of the colour that you are using.

Meditation

The bath is a very good place in which to meditate (see pages 140–41), so you can combine these two methods of colour healing. It would also help to visualize the effect you are trying to achieve (see pages 146–49). Or you can try breathing in the colour that you want to absorb (see pages 134–35). However, it is important to remain alert so that you do not drop off to sleep in the bath.

Temperature
Baths of colours at the red end of the spectrum will raise your temperature on a cold morning. Baths of colours at the blue end of the spectrum will cool you down on a hot day.

Warm end of spectrum

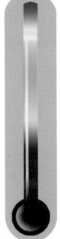

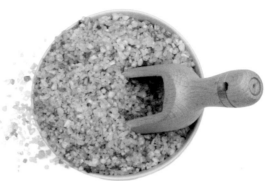

Bath salts
Pink bath salts will help you feel good about yourself and attract the warmth and love of others.

Cool end of spectrum

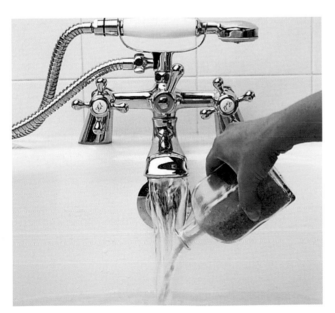

Blue, indigo & violet
A blue bath will help you unwind after a busy day and put your mind at rest. An indigo bath will help you escape from the everyday world and meditate on higher things. And a violet bath will inspire you to new heights of idealism in your work and life. All of these baths are best taken later in the day, when we are more inclined to relax.

Different Kinds of Colour Baths

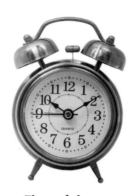

Time of day
Different colours of bath are suited to different times of the day or night.

Baths of colours that lie at the warm end of the spectrum are best taken in the morning, since they have a stimulating effect that will energize you for the day. You need to be particularly careful with red, however, because it is such a strong energy. Nevertheless, a red or an orange bath is a good treatment to take on a cold winter morning, since it will get the circulation going and help ward off colds and chills.

If your thinking is fuzzy or you find yourself unable to make a decision, you might want to add some yellow bath salts or a few drops of rosemary oil, which corresponds to yellow's colour frequency, to your bath to help stimulate and clear your mind. The yellow bath is definitely not one to take before you go to bed since it makes you very alert.

A green bath is an appropriate one to take in the summer, when you will be in harmony with the green of nature. It is good in the afternoon, when many of us tend to slow down after the bustle of the morning. Such a bath will refresh and relax you.

Evening baths

Baths of colours at the cool end of the spectrum are best taken in the evening since they have a sedative effect. Try adding some blue bath salts or a few drops of geranium essential oil to your bath, to help dissolve the stress and tensions of the day. Alternatively, several drops of patchouli oil will help you to reflect on your problems and come up with intuitive solutions to them. Lavender oil is particularly good for adding to a bath taken just before you go to bed. It relaxes you both physically and emotionally and will therefore help you sleep. It is also an antidepressant.

Cleansing the aura

From time to time it is a good idea
to take a bath to cleanse the aura. The
aura collects negative energies from
the environment and other people. Most
of us will be familiar with the experience
of feeling drained after being with certain
people – this is particularly true for healers
and other members of the helping
professions.

A turquoise bath is especially good for
cleansing the aura, as it strengthens the
immune system; white bath salts are also
good for this purpose. Even sprinkling
some ordinary sea salt into your bath
can help to renew your aura.

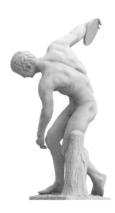

Aura-soma

The aura is the electromagnetic field surrounding the body. Soma comes from the Greek word for 'body'. The hyphen connecting the words indicates the relationship between the two.

AURA-SOMA
The name given to this particular form of colour healing revealed itself to Vicky Wall, a pharmacist and chiropodist, while she was meditating one day in 1984. Since then, aura-soma colour therapy has spread all over the world; thousands of people train to practise it and many more buy and use its products.

Balance bottles

Like other methods of colour healing, aura-soma works on the principle of balance and its distinctive bottles of coloured liquids are actually called 'the balance bottles'. The liquids come in two layers: the one on top consists of a mixture of oils and essences, while the one on the bottom is a solution of herbs. When shaken, the liquids combine into an emulsion that can be massaged into the skin. From there they are absorbed into the bloodstream and eventually by the organs of the body which, as we have seen, relate directly to the chakras (see pages 100–101).

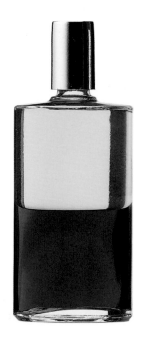
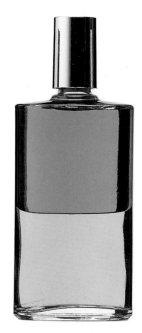

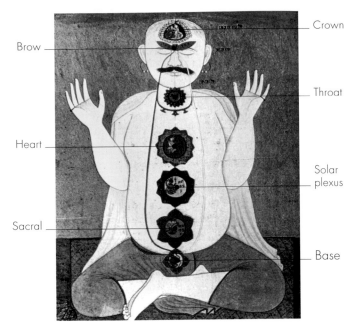

Brow —
Crown —
Throat —
Heart —
Solar plexus —
Sacral —
Base —

Chakras

For each of the major chakras there is a corresponding balance bottle, whose colours will help its energy to flow and restore balance to that part of the body. There are many other balance bottles and combinations of colours designed to treat specific ailments or enhance certain qualities.

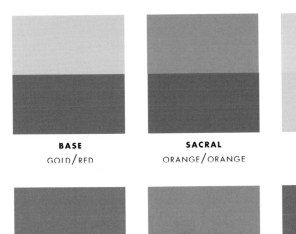

BASE
GOLD/RED

SACRAL
ORANGE/ORANGE

SOLAR PLEXUS
YELLOW/GOLD

HEART
BLUE/GREEN

THROAT
BLUE/BLUE

BROW
BLUE/PURPLE

CROWN
BLUE/PINK

Vicky Wall

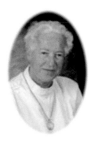

Vision
*The colours for the balance bottles came
to Vicky Wall in a vision one night.*

Vicky Wall was born the proverbial seventh child of a seventh child and from an early age she had psychic and mystical experiences. In her autobiography, *The Miracle of Colour Healing*, she tells the story of how she was scorned by her schoolfriends for remarking on the colours of their auras and how, on another occasion, she spontaneously healed the aunt of a classmate.

It was not until much later in her life that Vicky developed the mixture of oils and essences that went into aura-soma's beautiful coloured bottles. However, she saw her whole life as a preparation for that moment. Born into a Hassidic family in the early years of the twentieth century, as a girl Vicky was initiated into the healing properties of plants by her father, a master of the Qabalah, the ancient Jewish mystical tradition.

When she was in her fifties, Vicky suffered a major coronary, which was followed some years later by a massive haemorrhage that was to leave her blind as well. However, true to character, she regarded the consequent sharpening of all her senses and, in particular, her auric sight, or ability to see auras, as compensation for this.

'Divide the waters'

Vicky had been making up healing creams and lotions for years, but one night while meditating she was told to 'divide the waters'. She was mystified, but the next night the injunction was repeated. On the third night she got up and with little sense of what she was doing or how she did it, she made what came to be known as the balance bottles. These were of two layers of liquid, one lying upon the other, with the colour on the top usually of a different colour to the lower. The waters had indeed been divided.

Vicky was inspired to make many variations on her 'coloured jewels', as she called them, and today there are about one hundred balance oils. She also developed other ranges of plant essences and oils that she called pomanders and master quintessences. These differ from the balance oils in that they emit 'fragrant vapours', although colour is also the key to their healing properties.

The Balance Bottles

Each of the balance bottles has a name, such as 'Peace', 'New Beginning for Love' and so on, signifying its special quality. The different combinations of colours work on several levels – physical, mental, emotional and spiritual. Their effect is subtle, rather than dramatic, and they help us relate to our true selves.

AURA-SOMA COLOUR READING

The balance bottles work on many different levels – physical, emotional, mental and spiritual. When you go for an aura-soma colour reading, you will be asked to choose four bottles out of the whole range. You pick the ones you find yourself drawn to, using your intuition to guide you.

Choosing bottles

The first bottle represents your purpose in this incarnation, while the second shows the difficulties you have to overcome in order to achieve it. The third bottle stands for the here and now and shows how you are actually doing and the fourth reveals what the future has in store for you. Together they make up what Vicky Wall has called 'a mirror of your soul'.

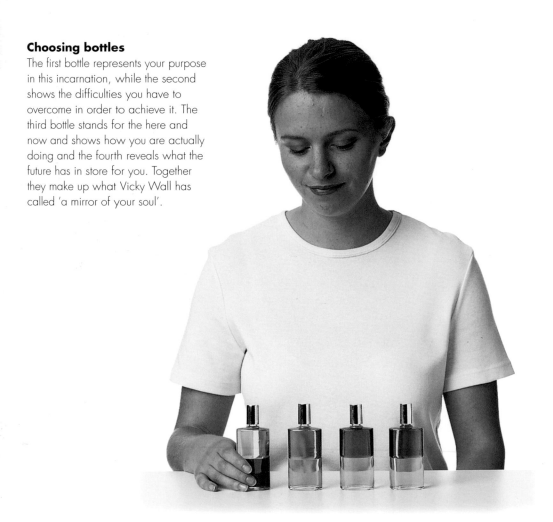

Discussing your choice

You will then discuss the chosen bottles with the aura-soma colour therapist, who will help you to relate the colours you have chosen to your physical and mental well-being, emotional state and soul's evolution. At this point you will be asked to shake the bottles vigorously, so that the two layers of liquid are well mixed. While you are doing this you are also putting some of your own energy into the contents, increasing their healing potential.

Shaking the bottles

If you are in a generally healthy state, the bubbles produced should settle quite quickly; if you are not, the effect will be cloudy and this can take some time to clear. The therapist will then advise you on how best to use the bottles. The methods you will be told to employ are likely to include rubbing the shaken mixture into your skin, so that you can absorb the energy of the colours. You can also just place the bottles strategically around your home or office, so that you benefit from their healing qualities just by looking at them or having them near you.

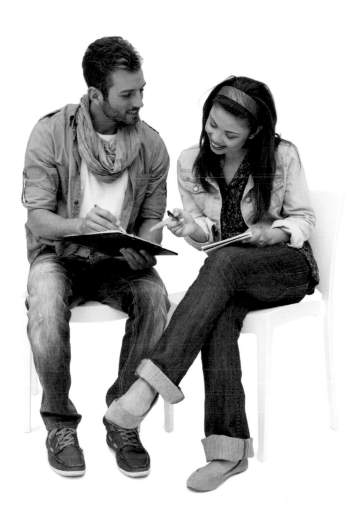

Crystals, Gems & Stones

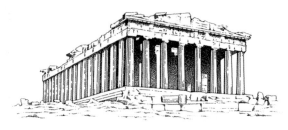

Ancient temples
In ancient times crystals were built into the very foundations of temples and other buildings.

Crystals, gems and stones are formed from the minerals that make up the Earth's crust and part of their appeal for humanity is their timelessness. Throughout history they have never ceased to fascinate humans and they have been prized for the status they bestow, the luck they are thought to bring and perhaps, above all, for their special healing properties. Ancient temples were built out of them, Egyptian pharaohs were buried with them and no modern state occasion would be complete without them. Crystals, gems and stones are part of human myth and legend, and some of them have become legends in their own right, such as the famous Koh-i-noor diamond, which weighs 108.8 carats

and literally means 'mountain of light'. The Koh-i-noor has a long and bloody history that goes back to the fourteenth century, but since the annexation of the Punjab in 1849 it has formed part of the British crown jewels.

Crystals

Crystals consist of millions of atoms and the density of these atoms is responsible for crystals' multi-faceted shapes. When heat or pressure is applied to a quartz crystal, the atomic structure is disturbed, producing a current of electricity oscillating from one end to the other. This process is known as piezoelectricity and in modern times has been applied in radio, television and satellite communications, as well as in technology requiring a high degree of precision. When the external application of pressure stops, the atoms rearrange themselves, so that the crystal is once more in balance. This shows, therefore, that crystals are both transmitters and receivers of energy, and it is thought that they can absorb and respond to our thoughts and emotions. They seem to have an ability to restore balance to a part of the body that is

experiencing disease or disharmony.
Crystals and gemstones have long been
used for this purpose in India where,
ground into a powder and mixed with
water or simply immersed in liquid and
placed in the sun, they are still prescribed
by doctors of Ayurvedic medicine.

Koh-i-noor Diamond

The Koh-i-noor diamond resides in the UK as
part of the crown of Queen Elizabeth the Queen
Mother. The crown was created when she
became Queen Consort in 1937. The diamond
was originally presented to Queen Victoria in
1849 and worn by her as a brooch and circlet.
On her death it became part of the crown jewels.

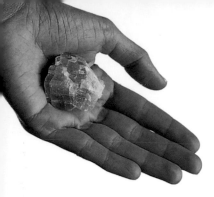

Right for you

Handling a crystal will help you decide if it is right for you.

CHOOSING A CRYSTAL

It is very important, when choosing a crystal for yourself, to follow your intuition and not to be swayed by what someone else thinks is right for you. Walking into a crystal shop or up to a stall selling crystals at an exhibition can be a bit mind-boggling at first, but if you focus on why you have come, you will find that a particular crystal will 'speak' to you. It will pick you out of the crowd, as it were, and that is the crystal for you.

Handling Your Crystal

Pick up the crystal you have chosen and hold it in the palm of your right hand (change this to the left one if you are left-handed) and see how it feels to you. Does it feel cool or warm? Does it make you tingle? You may not get any physical sensation at all, but still feel that it is right for you.

Many other people will probably have picked that crystal up and handled it before you chose it, so when you get home, you need to cleanse it of any negative energies that it may have absorbed. This can be done by taking a small bowl, preferably of glass or ceramic than of a synthetic material such as plastic, pouring some mineral or filtered water into it and then adding some sea salt. Then place the crystal into the bowl and let it stay there for as long as feels right to you.

If the crystal is for your own personal use, do not let anyone else handle it. Place it in a sunny spot on a windowsill or the top of a bookcase. Crystals, being creatures of the Earth like ourselves, need sunlight and air, although sometimes it's appropriate to keep them wrapped up in a piece of dark-coloured silk or other natural fabric to project them from negative influences. As you get to know your crystal, you will find out what it likes.

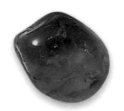

Ruby & garnet

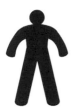

The ancient Egyptians massaged themselves with rubies and garnets to stimulate the cells of the body. Both stones were also thought to bring luck and good fortune.

Peridot

In ancient civilizations this brilliant stone was used to purify both the mind and the body. It aids the digestion and is particularly good for cleansing the liver.

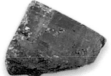

Amber & topaz

Both of these stones with their warm, golden hue will help to dissolve barriers in communicating with others when placed on the navel and solar plexus areas.

Amethyst

If you are a very emotional person, the amethyst will help you to stay in control. Placed between the eyebrows, it will also help activate the inner vision.

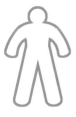
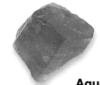

Quartz

The different kinds of quartz share the quality of breaking down negative patterns of behaviour, clearing the mind and generating positive energy.

Aquamarine

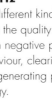

Associated with the sea, this stone is good for eliminating fluid from the body. It also helps with negative emotions, like anxiety and doubt

Crystal Healing

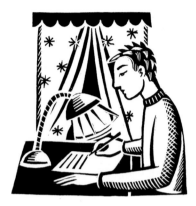

Relax or work
*Crystals can be placed around
the home or office to help you
either to relax or work.*

Part of the healing power of crystals derives from their colour. This is is important to bear in mind when you find yourself attracted to a particular stone because it may be its colour that is calling you.

If you find yourself drawn to one of the red stones – a garnet, carnelian or agate, for example – it may be that you are in need of some red energy, perhaps because you are anaemic or feeling listless, or your base chakra is not functioning well. The red stones motivate and energize us and are good for the circulation and sex drive. The king of the red stones, of course, is the ruby, which has the power to heal the spirit as well as the body.

Perhaps the best known of the orange stones is amber, the translucent fossil resin that sometimes contains trapped insects. Like its warm, glowing colour, it promotes emotional well-being and gives protection against negativity from within yourself and from external influences. Another stone with similar qualities to amber is topaz, which is good for shock and emotional trauma.

The yellow quartz, citrine, stimulates the mind and helps communication with others. It is a good stone to have in your study if you are writing a report or an article that calls for clarity of thought. If it is placed in your office it will help you to make decisions.

Green, blue, indigo & violet

Green is the colour of the heart chakra and green stones can help with problems of the heart, whether physical or emotional. Wearing an emerald or a jade pendant over your heart will help you to open up to others, without any fear or inhibition.

The sapphire comes in many colours, but the blue variety is perhaps the most highly valued. It is associated with the 'blue' attributes of truth, integrity and wisdom. Aquamarine promotes tranquility and peace and it also soothes fever, stings and burns. Its name comes from the Latin *aqua marina*, meaning seawater, and so it is also considered to bring luck to sailors and fishermen and to anyone making journeys by sea.

The stone that is most commonly associated with violet is amethyst. It has spiritually uplifting and transforming properties. Place one under your pillow at night to help you to sleep.

BioElectric Shield

The BioElectric Shield is a pendant containing quartz crystals, and is said to deflect harmful electromagnetic energy. Hillary Clinton, Cherie Blair and Steven Seagal have all worn one in the past.

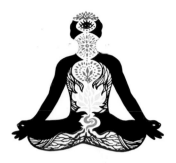

Ancient
The ancients practised colour breathing as a form of colour healing.

COLOUR BREATHING

This is one of the oldest methods of colour healing, which dates back to Atlantean times. It is also one of the simplest and cheapest as it doesn't involve any outlay at all. The key to it is the breath. This is what Hindus call *prana*, which is a Sanskrit word meaning 'the life-giving breath'.

Inhaling energy

Colour breathing is literally what it says – breathing in colour and then permeating the whole body with it, or directing it to a particular part of the body. One of the best times to practise it is at the beginning of the day – outside if possible if the weather allows and you have a garden or patio, inside if you do not, preferably in front of an open window. You may well want to do one or two stretching exercises first, to limber up and relax your body.

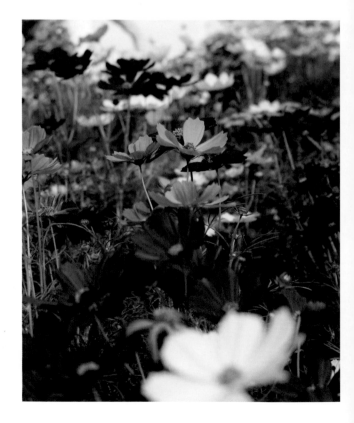

Fresh air
If you can, do your colour breathing outside, in the fresh air.

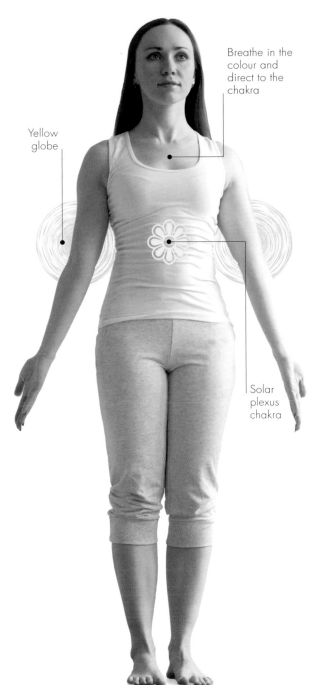

Breathe in the
colour and
direct to the
chakra

Yellow
globe

Solar
plexus
chakra

How to colour breathe

1 *Choose the colour that you want to
use – perhaps one of the warm colours
to energize you for the day ahead.*

2 *Stand with your feet a little apart,
arms stretched out to either side. Shut
your eyes if it helps you focus.*

3 *Visualize a globe of the colour in
front of you, behind you and to either
side of you. Now breathe it into the
corresponding chakra. If yellow, for
example, direct it to the solar plexus –
hold it, and then breathe out again –
this time without the colour, because
you have absorbed it.*

4 *Do the whole process again,
circulating the colour around the rest
of your body.*

Colour choice

You can use this method with any
colour or for each of the chakras,
one after the other, if you like. If you
choose one particular colour, you
may well find that you notice it more
than usual during the rest of the day.
Your environment, whether your home,
office or nearby park, will reinforce
it for you, in the clothes that people
wear, the colours of flowers and so on.

The Fourfold Breath

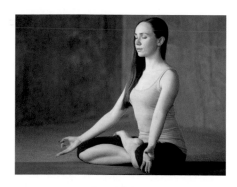

Practising
Before you start practising your breathing, make sure that you will not be disturbed.

Colour breathing combines the act of breathing with concentration on a colour. The energy of the colour you inhale can be directed to heal a chakra that may have absorbed negativity from your thoughts and actions and any part of the body.

If you are not accustomed to breathing in the way that is described on pages 134–35, you can practise doing it on its own at first, without the colour, until you are used to it.

Breathing sequence

1 Choose a quiet moment and lie or sit down in a room on your own, making sure that you are comfortable.

2 Breathe in slowly and deeply for a count of four, hold for a count of two and then breathe out again for a count of four.
3 When you breathe in, start right down in your belly, then let your diaphragm expand and finally fill your lungs with air.
4 When you breathe out, reverse the process, letting the chest contract first, then the diaphragm and finally the belly.
5 While you are getting the hang of this, it may help if you place your hand over your belly, so that you can feel it expanding and contracting.

Practise doing this until it feels natural to you, but be careful not to hyperventilate – most of us are shallow breathers and are not used to taking deep breaths. If you do find yourself feeling a little dizzy, just stop and breathe normally until you recover.

Environment

The beauty of colour breathing is that you can do it anywhere, combining the colour you breathe in with that in the environment. Try walking alongside a river or the sea, breathing in the colour blue; not only will the water energize you, but when combined with the colour blue, it will settle your mind, clearing it of mundane concerns and inspiring more spiritual thoughts.

Alternatively, as you walk over fields and through woods, breathe in the colour green, which is the colour of the grass beneath your feet and the leaves over your head. This will give you a deep feeling of harmony with your surroundings.

Affirmations

You can also practise your affirmations (see Chapter 2, pages 22–93) as you walk; as you breathe in the colour, say out loud (or silently in your mind if you prefer) the sentence that you have written for yourself. This will reinforce the positive attributes of the colour for you.

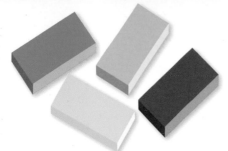

Colours
Breathing in certain colours will help rid your aura of anything negative. Gold, blue, turquoise and violet are the best colours to use for this.

THE CLEANSING BREATH
Just as you can take a colour bath to cleanse your aura (see pages 120–21), you can also use the breath to cleanse it. Like anything else, the aura can get polluted by habits such as drinking and smoking, stress, negative environments and negative people. The best colours to use to cleanse the aura are gold, blue, turquoise, violet or, if you prefer, white light.

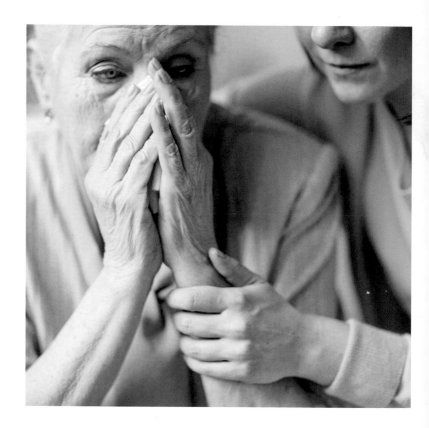

Helping people
If you help other people, then cleansing your aura should be part of your routine.

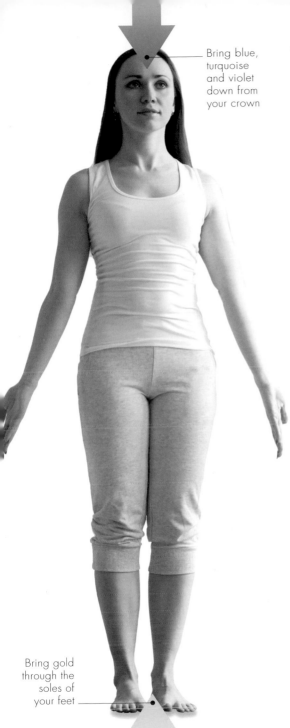

Bring blue, turquoise and violet down from your crown

Bring gold through the soles of your feet

Cleansing the aura

1 *Stand with your feet a little apart, with your arms hanging loosely by your sides.*

2 *Breathe in the colour that you have chosen. If it is gold, bring it up from beneath the soles of your feet, up through the chakras, one by one; if it is one of the other colours, bring it down from just above the crown of your head, again through the chakras.*

3 *As you breathe out, without the colour, imagine that you are expelling the tensions of the day, all the negative emotions and anything else that your aura may have collected that you want to get rid of. If you have chosen the first method, you can imagine the waste disappearing into the ether; if the second, being buried in the Earth.*

4 *Repeat the process until you are satisfied your aura is cleansed.*

Regular treatment

It is good to get into the habit of cleansing your aura regularly, particularly if you are a nurse or a therapist of some kind, as your work involves helping people who are ill or disturbed in some way. There are also people we meet in the course of everyday life who deplete our energy, leaving us feeling tired and low. If you feel this has happened to you, then just cleanse your aura in the way described, and then you can recharge it with one of the warmer, energetic colours.

Meditation

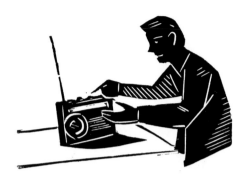

Peace & quiet
*It is important to have peace and quiet
if you are going to meditate.*

Meditation involves going within, to distance yourself from the distractions of the outer world and just to be with yourself – or *your self*, that vital inner part of you that it is so easy to lose touch with in a busy life revolving around home, work, family and friends.

To do this, you need silence, which many people in our busy, noisy modern world are so unused to that they feel unnerved by it. We are continually bombarded by various levels of background noise from things such as computers, TVs, mobile phones, traffic, telephones and so on. However, it is only when the clamour of external life has been tuned out that we can turn our attention inward to reflect, dream and meditate.

If you are not used to meditating, don't worry as you will soon get the hang of it. Like most things, it comes with practice.

Meditation basics
The important thing, first of all, is to make sure that you choose a time when you know you will not be disturbed by such things as your mobile phone going off, the doorbell, the demands of children or someone else walking into the room.

One thing you will notice when you start meditating is that your mind chatters away about all kinds of irrelevancies, such as what you are having for dinner, or what so-and-so said to you the other day. Just let these things pass through your mind without dwelling on them and you will find that after a while, as your internal focus grows, they fade into the background.

Meditating on colour
Meditating on colour is another age-old technique for self-healing. It allows you to focus on a particular chakra that may not be functioning well.

By meditating on the colour associated with a chakra, you can restore it to balance and harmony. Say, for example, that you feel you are in a rut, that your life is going along all right, but you are bored and are not having a lot of fun. By meditating on the colour orange you can regain your appetite for life, and this will help you to make the changes that will lead you to engage with it again. To find the best colour to meditate on, refer to Chapter 2 (see pages 22–93).

Meditation Benefits

Regular meditation can help improve a variety of conditions: headaches, migraines, anxiety, depression, asthma and breathing difficulties, insomnia, chronic pain, blood pressure problems, circulatory disorders, high blood pressure, stress-related disorders and muscular aches and pains. It improves awareness, concentration and emotional well-being.

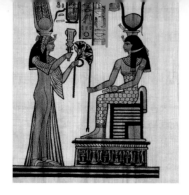

Energy flow
Sitting with a straight back and feet on the floor will help the energy flow through the chakras.

MEDITATING ON THE CHAKRAS
Sit down in a chair, with your feet on the floor, your back against the back of the chair and your hands resting on your thighs. This is known as the Egyptian position, after the pose of Egyptian pharaohs. Take a few moments to relax, making sure you are comfortable, before beginning your meditation.

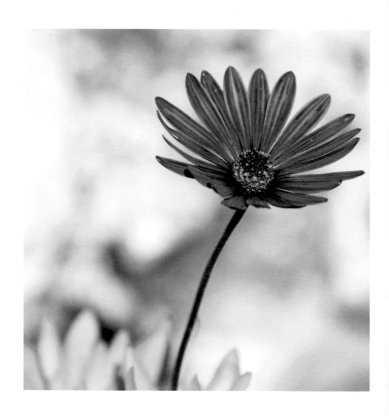

Closing the chakras
It is very important to remember to close your chakras when you have finished your meditation. Otherwise you will be vulnerable to external influences. View your chakras like flowers, with the petals folding inward to protect the centre. Then gently bring your awareness back to the present and, when you are ready, open your eyes.

Chakra meditation

1 *Close your eyes – this will help you to shut out the external world and focus inwardly.*

2 *Start breathing in the way described on pages 136–37, and, after two or three fourfold breaths, let your breathing return to normal. As you breathe, open your chakras one by on. If you are not used to doing this, imagine that they are flowers, opening up to the light.*

3 *Now focus on the centre of your chest, where the heart chakra is located. Imagine a ray of green light entering it from the side and filling it with love – for yourself, your loved ones, your neighbours, colleagues – even people that you do not particularly like or get along with.*

4 *Let the light radiate out through your upper chest, along your arms and into your hands. Allow yourself to bask in the peace and harmony that it brings, as you are opening your heart to your fellow human beings, with whom you are one. This is a particularly good meditation to do if you are feeling lonely or have recently been hurt in a relationship.*

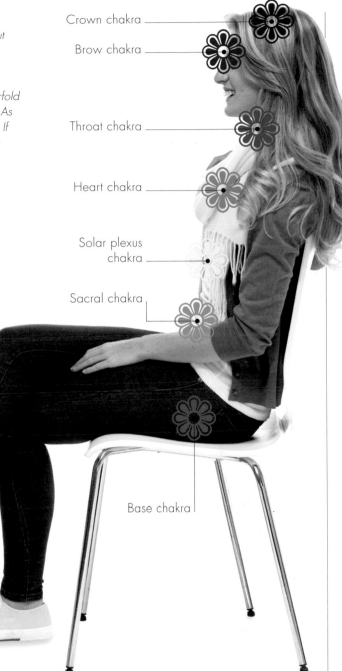

Crown chakra

Brow chakra

Throat chakra

Heart chakra

Solar plexus chakra

Sacral chakra

Base chakra

The Rainbow Meditation

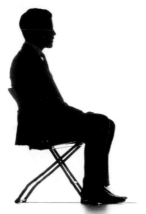

Red, orange & yellow
*Bring in the red, orange and yellow rays
from beneath the soles of your feet.*

The rainbow meditation is a wonderful way to start the day and you can combine it with colour breathing. Take up position and relax as described previously. Now take some deep breaths and open up your chakras (see pages 136–37 and 142–43). Then imagine the red ray rising – or breathe it in – from beneath the soles of your feet up to your base chakra, allowing the colour's energy and warmth to suffuse your whole body. (If you have heart trouble of any kind or you feel that red is too strong a colour for you, you can use the pink ray instead.)

Next bring the orange ray up to your sacral chakra and feel a sense of joy and vitality pervade your whole being. It is a new day and you look forward to what it brings. Now turn your attention to the yellow ray, allowing it to rise from beneath the soles of your feet to your solar plexus and then to spread throughout your body. As it does so, feel your mind quicken and awaken to the possibility of new ideas.

Moving through the rainbow

Now it is the turn of the green ray; imagine it entering the heart chakra horizontally, and, as it does so, feel it bringing you a sense of peace and fellowship with others. As you circulate the colour through your body, allow it to balance any part of you that feels out of kilter.

The blue, indigo and violet rays should be brought in from just above the crown of your head. Blue then goes to the throat chakra, first of all, to facilitate fluency of speech and also the wisdom to say what other people need to hear. Imagine as your breathe it in that the calmness of blue will stay with you throughout the busy day to come.

Now imagine the indigo ray lighting up your brow chakra, and as it does so, it brings you insight into your life and the intuition you need to navigate the day successfully.

Finally, beam the violet ray down into your crown chakra and feel its idealism pervading your consciousness, inspiring you to act for the highest good.

Remember to close your chakras when you have finished this process. You may also like to imagine yourself wearing a cloak of white light to protect yourself from negative energies throughout the day.

Regular Meditation

If you do this kind of meditation regularly, you may find that a particular colour comes to you as you prepare yourself. This is the one to take in, since you may need it for the day ahead.

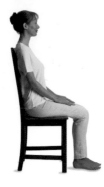

Techniques
Visualization uses the same relaxation and breathing techniques as meditation.

VISUALIZING COLOUR Here is a visualization that you might try for yourself sometime. First, take up position, relax and start breathing as you did for colour breathing and meditation. Next, open your chakras and then return your breathing to normal. Now, imagine that you are going for a walk through your favourite part of the countryside, and are leaving your everyday concerns behind. Already your heart feels lighter and there is a spring in your step.

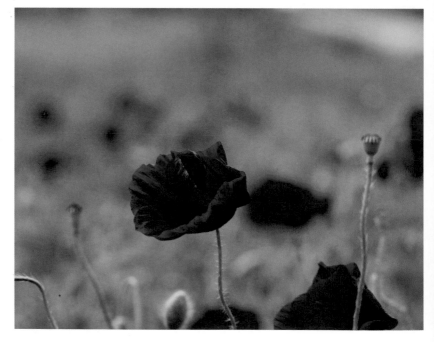

The visualization
1 *You now take a path off the road, leading down to a meadow whose lush green brings you a sense of peace. Red poppies are dotted among the tall grass and the sight of them lifts your spirits. With renewed energy you go on your way.*

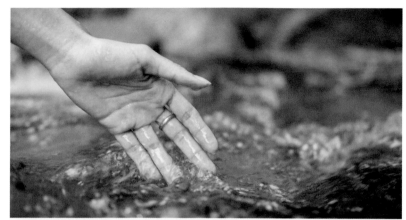

2 *You reach a gurgling brook. Gazing into its clear depths, you feel the cobwebs lifting from your mind. You dip a hand in the water and its coolness refreshes you.*

3 *A little way off you spot a shady copse. You lie under a tree there, on ground dappled with warm, golden sunlight.*

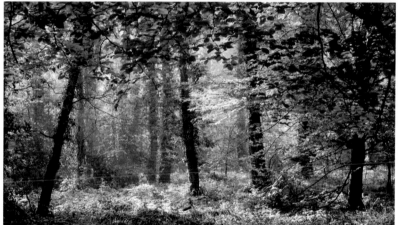

4 *A clump of harebells grows by your head. Idly you daydream. In this relaxed state, the answer to a problem that has been worrying you may come into your mind.*

5 *You make your way back to the spot where you joined the road, and begin to close down your chakras. In your own time bring yourself back to your real surroundings and open your eyes. You can do this visualization any time, anywhere – such as in the office.*

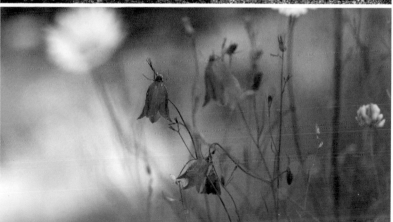

Visualization

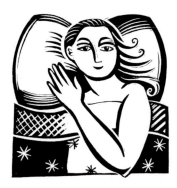

Going to sleep
Before you go to sleep at night, train your mind to visualize the day's events and encounters.

Visualization is a similar process to meditation, except that it involves seeing or creating pictures with the inner eye, which is why it is sometimes known as creative visualization. This process comes more easily to some people than to others. Ask them what they had for lunch, and on to the inner screen of their mind will immediately flash a picture of a bowl of soup and a sandwich. You may be the type of person who senses things more, feels or even hears them. However, with practice, even if you do not consider yourself to be a particularly visual person, you can train your mind to visualize, using your powers of observation and recall.

Bedtime

At night, before you go to sleep, go over the day, but instead of mulling over the problems that arose, think of the places that you went to or the people that you met and try and recall them in as much detail as possible. If you are recalling a person, then try to remember what they were wearing. How did they have their hair? And what were they carrying? If you practise this often enough, you are likely to find that you have only to think of a name for a picture to come to mind.

I spy with my little eye

Can you remember playing 'I spy with my little eye' as a child, in the back of the car or on a train journey? Try it again the next time that you are travelling and have time to kill. Look out of the window at the landscape, at the buildings that are passing by and note any special features that they have. Later on, try and recall what you have seen in as much detail as possible.

What you are doing with this process is training the mind to file away pictures for future use. Eventually you will get to the point where you will be able to summon

up pictures from your mind's very own
'picture library' at will, simply by recalling
a name or a place. This is obviously a
very useful ability to have if you go on the
holiday of a lifetime and want to go back.
All you have to do is file away the picture
of the turquoise sea, the empty beach or
the mountain top and you can go back
whenever you wish.

Mind Games

Visualization can be done any time and
anywhere. That way, wherever you are and
whatever the weather, you can always go
to your own special place.

You can do it in the office during your lunch hour,
perhaps using it to escape from a dark winter's
day to a sun-drenched Mediterranean scene.
Or you can visualize a favourite walk.

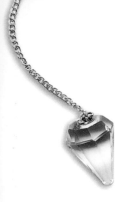

Your own needs
You can combine different colour healing methods to suit your own needs and tastes.

COMBINING METHODS
Visualization, meditation and colour breathing can all be enhanced by other methods of colour healing, for example, crystal healing. A coloured cloth is particularly useful if you have difficulty envisaging a colour. Put it in front of you and look at it for a few moments. Then, the mental image will stay with you when you close your eyes.

Revitalizing

If you do decide to use coloured cloth it is best to use pure silk or cotton, because they are natural fabrics and are therefore better conductors of the vibration of the colour. If you have been working very hard and you feel physically run down and have difficulty motivating yourself, try meditating on the positive attributes of the colour red – energy, will, enthusiasm – or visualize red going into your base chakra. It will help if you drape a piece of red cloth, such as a shawl or a scarf, over your pelvis. If you have a heart problem, of course, you should avoid using red. When in doubt, leave red out.

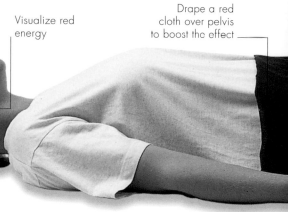

Visualize red energy

Drape a red cloth over pelvis to boost the effect

Raising self-esteem

You can also use crystals in a similar way. If, for example, you are not feeling particularly good about yourself – perhaps you are estranged from someone or are not getting the recognition that you feel you deserve at work – then try using a piece of rose quartz to aid a meditation on the colour pink. This is the colour of love and it will help to raise your self-esteem as well as attract the love of others.

ROSE QUARTZ

Relaxing

Alternatively, if perhaps you are in an agitated state of mind and cannot settle down to an urgent task, try lying down on the floor and covering yourself with a blue sheet or blanket. Breathe in the colour blue, firstly to your throat chakra and then throughout your head. Continue until you feel your mind has come to rest and you have your powers of concentration back.

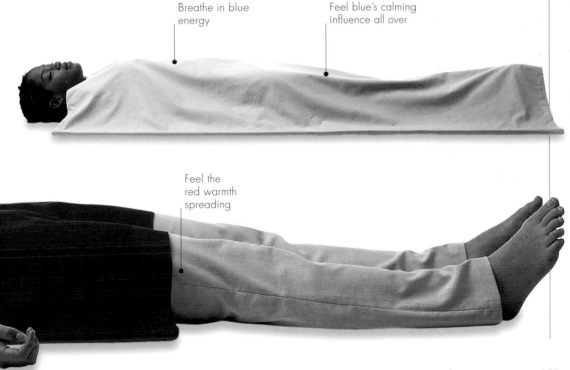

Breathe in blue energy

Feel blue's calming influence all over

Feel the red warmth spreading

Absent Healing

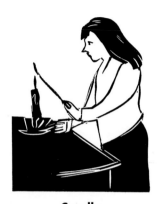

Candle
Lighting a candle in the same colour can aid the sending of healing.

Absent healing is exactly what it says – it is healing someone in their absence, by means of meditation or visualization. In the case of colour, it involves mentally transmitting colour to the other person. It is a good idea for the two people involved to link up, by agreeing on a mutually convenient time for the healing to take place. Then the person who is being healed by this method can be open to receiving it. You can also link in other ways. It is a good idea for both people to light a candle of the colour being used in the healing.

Having faith

You can send healing to someone even if you do not link up, although it is probably more effective if you do. You should be careful, though, of sending healing to someone who does not want it or does not believe in it. They may not welcome it, or may think it intrusive, even if they are ill or unhappy. Absent healing works best when someone asks for it or agrees to it. It helps, too, if they are open to the process; a sceptical attitude can block the healing.

Creating what we think

If you believe that absent healing will work, there is a very good chance that it will. We tend to create what we think in our lives, which is why positive thinking is so important. If we go around with negative expectations of what will happen to us, our worst fears are likely to be fulfilled. If, on the other hand, we believe that things will turn out for the best, then we are likely to attract more positive experiences. As the saying goes, 'it's all in the mind'.

Sometimes the recipient of the absent healing may be too ill or depressed to actively cooperate with you. However, they may still feel the effect of the colour and just knowing that someone else is thinking of them and doing something to help them, even if it is from a distance, can be a form of healing in itself.

Radionics

This complementary therapy is also a form of absent healing. Developed in the United States in the 1920s by Albert Abrams, radionics relies on using an instrument called a 'black box' to analyse the vibratory patterns of a 'witness' (an item belonging to the patient, such as a lock of hair or drop of blood), to diagnose health problems.

The therapists then find out the best treatment (many radionics practitioners use colour therapy) and transmit healing radiations through the witness. The treatment given follows holistic principles, treating all aspects of the patient's physical, mental and emotional state. Radionics is a controversial therapy, though adherents claim to have treated many ailments successfully.

SENDING COLOUR HEALING
If you wish to send a healing colour to someone else, then prepare yourself in the same way as for meditation or visualization, taking deep breaths to relax the body and still the mind. Then picture the person you want to send healing to in your mind's eye; you may well find yourself 'tuning in' to them or 'feeling' their presence. Use a photograph of them if it helps you to concentrate.

Sending healing

1 *Visualize the person to whom you are sending the healing or use a photograph of them if it helps you focus.*

2 *Open your chakras – ideally the other person should do the same – and bring in the colour needed. You might be focusing on a specific condition or emotional state, or be doing this just for overall well-being. Refer to pages 22–93 if you are in any doubt about which colour to use. You can also dowse for the colour needed, or simply send white light, which of course contains all the colours of the spectrum.*

3 *Imagine the colour radiating out from you to the other person. Beam it onto them like a laser, so that they are bathed in colour; or direct it to a particular part of their body where you know they are experiencing pain or discomfort. Golden yellow is a good colour to send – they will take from it what they need. Don't forget to close down your chakras when you have finished.*

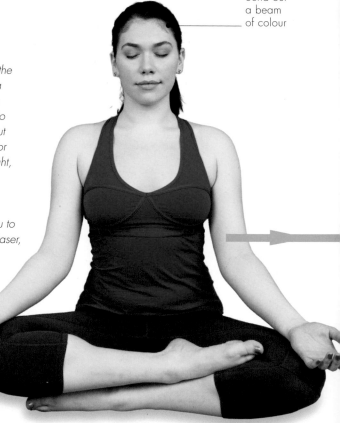

Send out a beam of colour

Receiving healing

If you have linked up with each other, then the other person can also imagine the colour being sent to them and this will aid the healing process. The whole session need not take very long; with practice, you will know when to stop and may even feel when the other person has had as much as they need. If they are going through a particularly bad time in their life, or are suffering from some kind of ongoing illness, you can make a regular appointment with them and send healing colour each time.

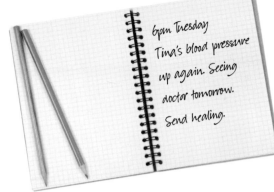

6pm Tuesday
Tina's blood pressure
up again. Seeing
doctor tomorrow.
Send healing.

Regular healing

The other person may want you to send healing to them on a regular basis.

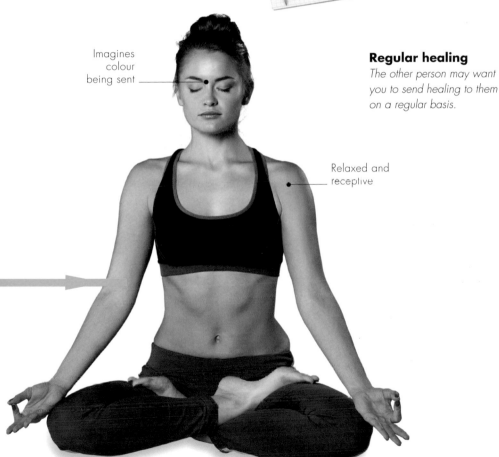

Imagines colour being sent

Relaxed and receptive

The Laying On of Hands

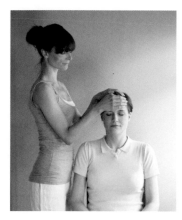

Healing process
Touching someone with your hands is a very effective part of the colour healing process.

In this form of healing the hands of one person are used to channel colour to another person. We all unconsciously use our hands for healing ourselves and others. Instinctively we put out a hand to soothe and comfort someone in pain or distress. If we ourselves have a headache or a stomach pain, we immediately put a hand on the spot without even thinking about it, while if someone we know is upset then we often react by laying a hand on them or putting an arm around them. Human touch has great healing power.

Preparation

If you are the one who will be doing the healing, then it is important for you to prepare yourself as you would for meditation or visualization. You should also make sure that your hands are warm before laying them on someone else. The recipient should sit or lie down in a position in which they feel comfortable and close their eyes, to help them relax. Then place your right hand over their solar plexus and your left over the chakra that corresponds to the part of their body where the pain or the problem is. Visualize the colour that is needed and imagine it flowing down your arm and into your right hand. It will then circulate through the other person's nervous system, and will finally complete the circuit at your left hand.

Colours to use

You may wish to use one of the blue colours because the other person is feeling stressed and is not sleeping well or is suffering from tension headaches. If, however, their physical vitality is low and they are lacking in confidence, then use red/orange. Use yellow if they are depressed or green if they have difficulty in relating to other people. Again, if you are not sure what colour to use, refer to the section on Chapter 2 (see pages 22–93).

When you become adept at this kind of colour healing, you will know when the circuit has been completed and the right moment at which you should withdraw your left hand. Once you have taken it off, you should then shake it vigorously, to get rid of any negative vibrations that you may have picked up. It is also important to wash your hands after every treatment to make sure that no residue is left.

Conviction

It is important that the recipient of healing is open to the power of the laying on of hands, and the ability of the healer to channel healing colour energies. Without this openness to the process on the part of the recipient, the chances of a successful outcome are reduced.

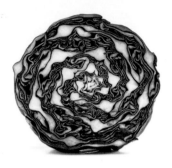

Food colour
*The colour of food is
one of the reasons we
are drawn to it.*

COLOUR YOU EAT
Colour is one of the attributes of food, along with aroma, texture and taste, that stimulates our appetite and gets us salivating. What's more, we often instinctively choose to eat food for the properties associated with its colour; for example, we eat oranges as a tonic when we have a cold, and red meat if we need an energy boost when we are feeling tired or have physical work to do.

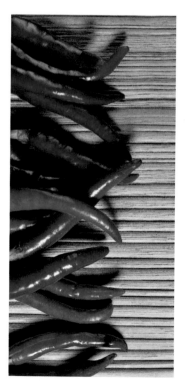

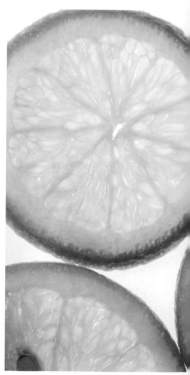

Nutrients
The colour of food also describes the nutrients that it contains; the vitamins and minerals that we need for healthy living. Once we know what these are, we can tailor our diet to what our bodies need on a day-to-day basis. It is a known fact that what we eat is a major contributing factor to good or ill health; and that some foods should be avoided if we are suffering from certain conditions, while others can be sought out for their healing properties.

A balanced diet

There are many different kinds of diets, some of them aimed at those who want to lose weight, others designed to alleviate specific conditions like cancer or arthritis. But if you adhere to a diet that includes food from each of the main groups – carbohydrates, fruit and vegetables, meat, fish and other proteins and some fats – in varying proportions, you will be ingesting all the colours of the spectrum.

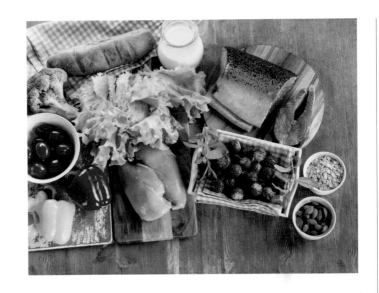

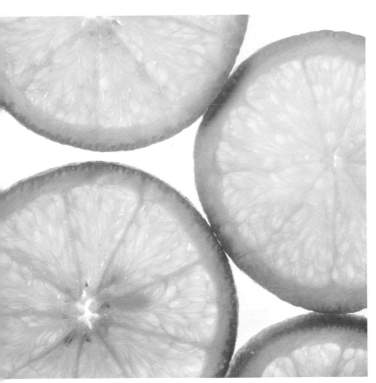

Seasonal variations

There will be times when you need to eat more of one kind of food than another, depending on the season, the weather and your own health, stress level or mood. The following pages are designed to help you pinpoint, using colour, the foods that you need for particular conditions or states of mind.

What Colour Do You Eat?

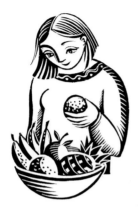

Looking at food
Look at the colour of the food that you eat – is it the colour that you need?

The questionnaire on the opposite page is designed to make you think carefully about the colours of the food that you eat, so take a few moments with a pen and paper to answer it. If you discover there is a colour missing from your fruit bowl or vegetable rack, you will need to consider the properties it possesses (refer to Chapter 2 on pages 22–93 if you need to refresh your memory). The absence of a colour and lack of a nutrient may be causing physical, mental or emotional problems.

Missing colours

If the questionnaire reveals that a certain colour tends not to feature in the food that you normally eat, does the missing colour relate to a particular complaint that you have? Do you, for example, tire easily or suffer from anaemia? It may be that there is not enough red food in your diet.

Red food contains iron and you may need to increase your consumption of liver and kidney, for example. If these foods are distasteful to you, you can substitute them with spinach or watercress, which also contain iron. You may find that you sometimes get a sudden craving for these foods – this is a sure sign that your body is out of balance and needs the nutrients that they contain.

The colour you eat the most

Think about the properties of the colour that you eat the most – work out which specific property you feel you need and why. Do the same thing for all the food you normally eat, and that way, from the colour alone, you will get a very good idea of whether your diet is balanced or not. If you feel it isn't, then you may

need to include more green food in
your diet – this will help you to counter
any lack or excess.

While colour can be a helpful guide to
establishing which foods you need to eat
more of, if you are in any doubt about your
nutritional requirements, it is best to consult
your doctor or a qualified dietician.

Questionnaire

What is the colour of your favourite food?

What food don't you like and what colour is it?

When you look in your vegetable rack, what colours do you see?

When you look in your fruit bowl, what colours do you see?

What colours are missing from both?

If you sometimes eat food on impulse, is it often of a specific colour?

If you suffer from a particular condition, do you eat special food for it? If so, what colour is it?

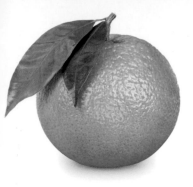

Feeling good
While your diet should contain a proportion of red, orange and yellow food, too much can lead to an excess of energy.

RED, ORANGE & YELLOW FOOD
Red, orange and yellow foods stimulate and energize our systems, cleanse and purify the blood and boost our immune levels. They also earth us, helping us to root in the physical world and engage positively with life. We need them to recharge our batteries and to keep infection and disease at bay.

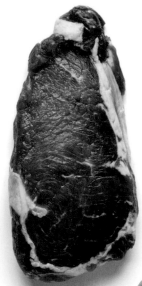

RED MEAT

Red food
Red food has already been mentioned as being important because it contains iron (see pages 160–61), essential for the formation of red blood cells and for keeping energy levels up. Even a mild deficiency of this mineral can lead to reduced work capacity and low resistance to disease.

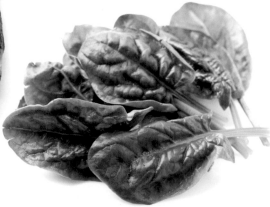

Iron intake
If you are a vegetarian, eat plenty of green leafy vegetables to replace the red meat you have given up. These foods are categorized as 'red' because they are also rich in iron.

SPINACH

Orange food

Orange food is associated with health and vitality, and in particular the all-important vitamin C, which is essential for overall good health. This vitamin can be found in citrus fruit. Carrots, another common orange food, contain beta-carotene, a major antioxidant that helps protect our defence system against air pollution. Honey, which is also an orange food, is good for the immune system.

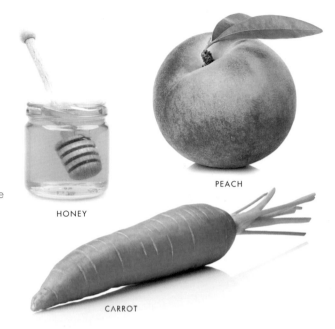

HONEY

PEACH

CARROT

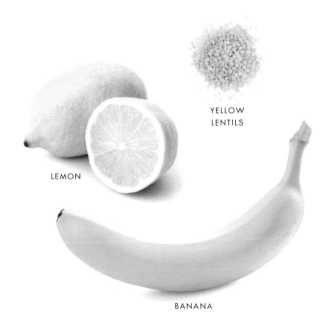

YELLOW
LENTILS

LEMON

BANANA

Yellow food

Yellow food is important for the efficient functioning of the digestive system and for detoxifying the body in general. It's also good for the nervous system and the mental faculties, including reasoning, memory and the ability to concentrate. Bananas, for example, one of the commonest yellow foods, are rich in potassium, and a deficiency in this mineral can lead to mental confusion and tiredness.

Cooking with Red

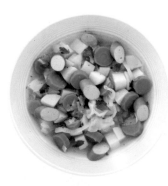

Warming

Red, orange and yellow food helps to warm and invigorate us as well as make us feel good.

f you are lacking red, orange or yellow energy, it's quite easy to introduce it into your diet. The foods listed below will give you some ideas.

Red foods

- Tomatoes, red peppers, red cabbage, beetroot, red chillies, kidney beans, watercress, leafy dark green vegetables (these contain iron which qualifies them for this section).
- Black and white pepper, ginger, cayenne pepper, rosemary, red sage.
- Red meat (do not eat to excess).
- Cherries, plums, rhubarb, apples, raspberries, strawberries, redcurrants.

Orange foods

- Pumpkin, squash, swede, carrots, orange peppers.
- Coriander seeds, cumin.
- Orange lentils, egg yolks.
- Oranges, tangerines, peaches, apricots, nectarines, mangoes, pawpaws, melons.

Yellow foods

- Sweetcorn, squash, yellow peppers.
- Saffron, cinnamon, lemongrass, dill, caraway.
- Yellow lentils, butter, oils, nuts, seeds, wholegrains.
- Pineapples, lemons, bananas, grapefruit.

Recipe

Autumn stew has been chosen for its red, orange and yellow ingredients. It is a very warming, comforting and energizing dish to eat as the colder days approach.

Autumn Stew

Serves two to three

INGREDIENTS

Half a red pepper, chopped

1 can chopped tomatoes

1 red chilli, de-seeded and cut into small pieces

250g (8oz) split red lentils

half a medium-sized swede,
peeled and cut into small pieces

3 medium-sized carrots, peeled and sliced

2 potatoes, peeled and cubed

1 medium-sized onion, sliced

3 cloves garlic (or to taste)

550ml (1pt) water

3.75 ml (¾ teaspoon) turmeric

5ml (1 teaspoon) cumin seeds

5ml (1 teaspoon) coriander seeds

1 dozen juniper berries

1 banana, sliced, as garnish

15ml (1 tablespoon) sunflower/olive oil

METHOD

Cover the lentils with cold water in a large casserole dish, then bring to a boil and cook for 10 minutes, skimming the surface as necessary. Put the lid on and simmer for 15–20 minutes until the lentils are a thick mush and all the liquid is absorbed. While the lentils are cooking, prepare the pepper, chilli, swede, carrots, potatoes, onion and garlic. Then fry the vegetables in a separate pan in oil for 3–4 minutes, turning them all the time.

When the lentils are ready, ladle in the vegetables together with the chopped tomatoes and add the cumin and coriander seeds as well as the juniper berries. Simmer the mixture gently for about an hour with the lid on until the vegetables are cooked, but not too soft.

Serve the dish garnished with a sliced banana. Autumn stew is usually enough on its own, but may be eaten with boiled rice, flavoured with 3.75ml (¾ tsp) of turmeric, as desired.

Tomatoes contain a significant amount of vitamin E, which may guard against cancer and heart disease; red pepper is high in vitamins C and E, and beta-carotene.

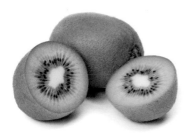

Healthy
It's difficult to imagine that you could eat too much green food since it's essentially so healthy. But it does need to be combined with food of other colours for an optimum healthy diet.

GREEN FOOD
Green is the colour of nature and so we view green food, such as salads, vegetables, fruit and herbs as natural and healthy. These contain many of the vitamins and minerals that are necessary to keep our bodies in balance, which is another property of green. It's now widely accepted that a healthy diet should include at least five portions of fresh fruit and vegetables a day.

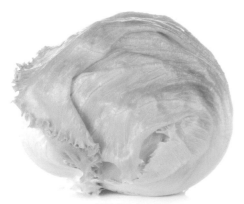

ICEBERG LETTUCE

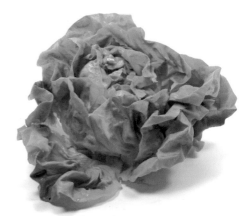

ROUND LETTUCE

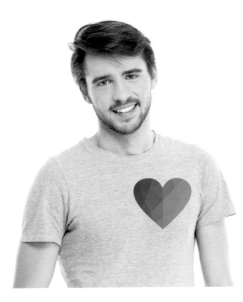

Hearty food

Green is also the colour that relates to the heart, and many green foods actually help to prevent heart disease. One of the causes of the disease is a diet low in the antioxidants vitamins C and E and beta-carotene. Green leafy vegetables are a particularly rich source of these. Lettuce is a good choice. It's best to buy organically grown if possible, since a lettuce's large expanse of leaf makes it particularly vulnerable to the chemicals that are used in fertilizers and pesticides. Therefore, if you do buy non-organic varieties always rinse them well before eating. Do not throw away the outer leaves, since these contain higher levels of vitamins than the inner leaves. The packets of lettuce leaves that are ready-washed and torn, although convenient, have already lost much of their goodness.

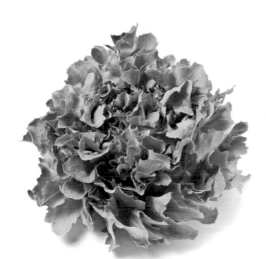

CURLY LEAF LETTUCE

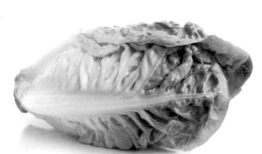

LITTLE GEM LETTUCE

Cooking with Green

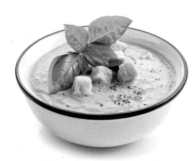

Vitamins & minerals
Green food is full of the vitamins and minerals we need for a healthy diet.

G reen foods are good for the heart; they also lower blood pressure, relieve stress and tension, alleviate headaches and help with emotional problems. Green is nature's balancing force, so foods of this colour are particularly good for bringing the body into harmony.

Green foods
- Cabbage, lettuce, green peppers, courgettes, peas, celery, artichokes, green beans, broccoli, cucumber, avocado, watercress, asparagus.
- Parsley, tarragon, alfalfa, mint, coriander, basil, chives.
- Green lentils, neutral foods including natural yoghurt and tofu.

- Apples, pears, kiwi fruit, limes, grapes, gooseberries, greengages.

Recipe
Watercress is a deep rich green and it is one of the healthiest foods we can eat. It contains particularly high levels of antioxidants – vitamins C, E and carotenes – as well as iron and potassium. This delicate, fragile little plant helps to reduce the risk of cancer, prevent infection and counter anaemia. It has a pungent peppery flavour and does not keep well, so is best used fresh. Try and obtain it from a watercress farm, since wild watercress is known to harbour parasites.

Other green ingredients in this recipe include aromatic chives and fennel, which has feathery fronds and a clean, fresh smell of aniseed. Fennel is particularly good for relieving colic and flatulence.

Watercress Soup

Serves two to three

INGREDIENTS

2 large bunches of fresh watercress, de-stalked

450–675g (1–1½lb) potatoes, peeled and chopped

50g (2oz) of butter or 15ml (1 tablespoon) extra virgin olive oil

850ml (1½pt) vegetable stock

150ml (¼pt) soured cream

4 large spring onions, finely chopped

handful of chives
and a few chopped fennel leaves

squeeze of lemon

salt and freshly ground pepper to taste

METHOD

De-stalk and chop the fresh watercress; peel and chop the potatoes and spring onions. Melt the butter or heat the olive oil in a heavy saucepan or casserole dish, then add the spring onions, potatoes and watercress, stirring until they are well coated with the butter or oil. Add salt, cover and let the vegetables sweat over a low heat for about 15–20 minutes, stirring periodically.

Add the stock, bring to simmering point and simmer, covered, for about 10–15 minutes until the vegetables are tender. Remove from the heat, allow to cool, and then liquidize for a short period only, to keep the texture slightly rough and not too glossy. Return to the saucepan, stir in the cream, add a squeeze of lemon and check the seasoning – very little pepper is needed.

Serve the soup either hot or cold, garnished with chives and fennel leaves.

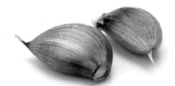

Inspiration
*Blue, indigo and violet
food is particularly good
to eat if you are lacking
in inspiration.*

BLUE, INDIGO & VIOLET FOOD
There is not such an abundance of blue, indigo and violet food as there is of other coloured food, but it still forms an important part of a healthy diet. It is the counter to red, orange and yellow food and it therefore cools and calms; it is also nourishing for the nervous system, brain and the higher mental faculties.

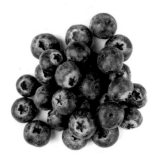

BLUEBERRIES

Brain food
This kind of food includes blue- and blackberries, purple-topped vegetables such as some varieties of broccoli, and red cabbage and onions. With the colour violet, we are coming around the colour wheel toward red again, so purple food is also energizing, particularly mentally.

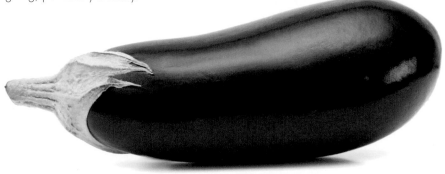

AUBERGINE

Sun ripened

Black or purplish-black grapes are one of the fruits that are included in this group of food. They are ripened on the vine, so when we eat them we are directly absorbing the rays of the sun. This also applies to other fruit and vegetables that are grown above ground. These should be eaten with their skins on, because this is the part that is exposed to the sun.

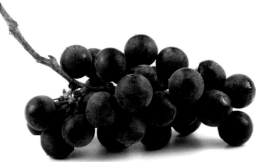

BLACK GRAPES

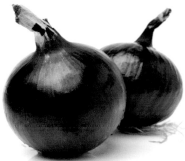

PURPLE-SKINNED ONIONS

Blue fish

Blue, indigo and violet food also includes some fish, for example oily fish like mackerel and sardines, which have a bluish tinge to their scales. The benefits of this kind of fish have been well established by extensive research. Oily fish contains omega-3 fatty acids, which help to prevent heart disease and relieve rheumatoid arthritis. They are also high in vitamin D, which the body needs in order to absorb calcium, which is vital for bone growth.

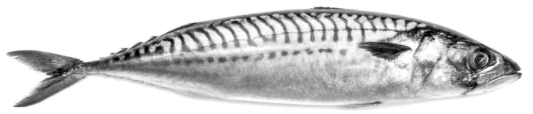

MACKEREL

Cooking with Blue

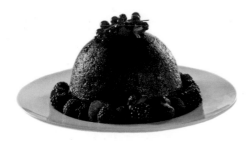

Healthy desserts

*Even desserts can be healthy
if they contain ingredients with
vitamins that we need.*

It is particularly good to introduce blue,
indigo and violet food into your diet if
you have been through a very stressful
time and need to slow down; or if you
want to withdraw from the busy outer
world for a while.

Blue foods are cooling and soothing,
sedative, antiseptic, anti-fungal and
bactericidal. Indigo foods too are
sedative; they also help with digestion,
purify and stabilize. Violet foods are
good for nervous disorders, rheumatism
and bladder troubles.

Blue, indigo & violet foods

- Purple-leaved lettuce, aubergines,
  sea vegetables, purple broccoli,
  mushrooms, black olives.
- Blue sage, juniper berries.
- Black beans, black soybeans.
- Black grapes, blueberries, plums,
  bilberries, blackberries, prunes, black
  cherries, raisins and currants.

Recipe

The berries that constitute the main
ingredient of this scrumptious Blue Summer
Pudding are rich in vitamins and high in
antioxidants. Blackberries are an excellent
source of vitamin E, while blueberries
are good for the eyesight and, like
blackcurrants, help to prevent infections
of the urinary tract. Blackcurrants also
contain a high level of vitamin C.

To make the dish even more fun, you
can make the cream blue by adding blue
colouring to it, or, more exotically, blue
curaçao. Add blue food colouring very
sparingly. Finally, decorate the pudding
with blue flowers.

Blue Summer Pudding

Serves two to three

INGREDIENTS

250g (9oz) blueberries

125g (5oz) blackberries

125g (5oz) blackcurrants

100g (4oz) caster sugar

several medium slices
of one-day-old white bread

275ml (½pt) double cream

several drops of blue colouring, or
8–15ml (½–1 tablespoon) blue curaçao

edible blue flowers

METHOD

Rinse the fruit and place it in a large saucepan with the sugar and 8–15ml (½–1 tablespoon) of water to stop it from sticking to the bottom of the pan before the juice has been released. Cook gently for 4–5 minutes until the sugar melts and the juice runs – do not leave it for any longer or the fruit will get too mushy. Save the juice and put it to one side.

Cut the crusts off of the bread and line the bottom and the sides of a 600–850ml (1–1½pt) pudding basin or souffle dish, with the slices, slightly overlapping them and pressing them together to seal the dish completely. Add the fruit, then make a lid with more bread, again sealing the edges carefully all around. Place a saucer or small plate over the top to fit inside the rim of the bowl, so the fruit can be pressed down. Add 1.4kg (3lb) or 1.8kg (4lb) weights on top of the plate and refrigerate the dish overnight.

Turn the pudding out and brush the bread with the saved fruit juice to cover any remaining white patches. Decorate the top with candied violets, edible blue flowers such as lavender, borage, cornflowers or pansies. Finally, add the blue colouring or blue curaçao to the cream and serve.

THE COLOUR OF YOUR
ENVIRONMENT

Colour is personal; the clothes we wear and the colour schemes of our homes and gardens all say a great deal about us. They indicate the state of our health, our mind and describe our personalities. It is important to surround ourselves with colours to which we are attracted, so that we feel in tune with, and supported by, our environment. It's also important to recognize that our need for colour changes as we ourselves change; while we may always have a favourite colour, there will be times when we have a sudden urge to redecorate a room or buy an article of clothing in a colour that normally we would avoid. This section of the book is designed to increase your awareness of what colour you are most drawn to at any given time and to help you change the colour of your environment to reflect that.

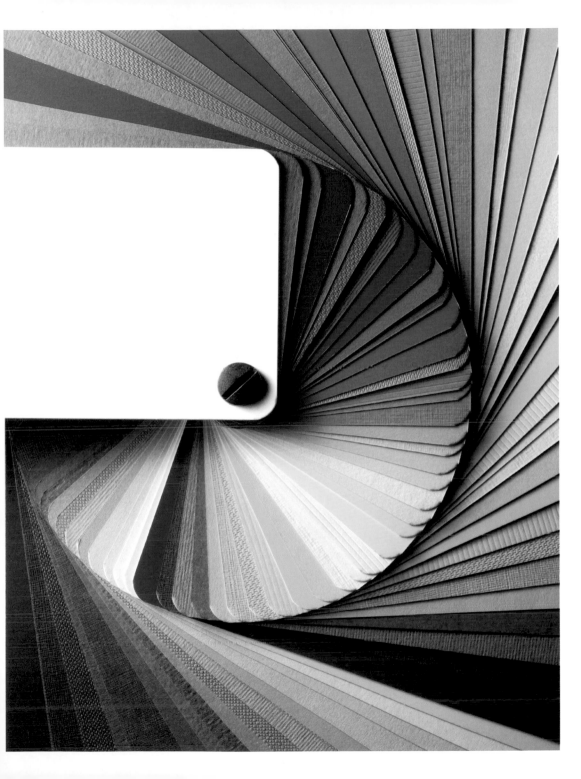

Uniform Colour

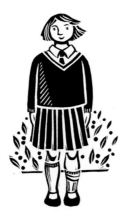

Uniformity
Most school uniforms are in the colours of conformity: blue, grey, brown and black.

Throughout history the properties of colour have been used in the form of dress in order to reinforce people in their traditional roles in society. Royalty, high-ranking members of the clergy and the judiciary, for example, have habitually donned purple, the colour of nobility, dignity and the highest form of self-expression. The colour of uniforms of all kinds indicates the qualities needed in their work by the people who wear them.

Red, for example, the colour of courage, action and aggression, has always been favoured by the military, particularly for show. It is also the colour of the blood that the fighting man spills. Blue, the colour of the sea, is the colour of naval uniforms, to the extent that navy blue is a colour in itself. Grey, or blue-grey, is the colour of the Royal Air Force uniform and is also the colour of the aircraft its pilots fly as well as the skies they fly through. We can tell, just by looking at the colour of the uniforms that these people wear, which roles they have and the qualities they need in order to perform them well.

Black, the colour of authority and power, is worn by the police, who have to enforce the law against the criminal element of society; it is also the colour of the habits worn by some religious orders, and here black carries the meaning of shutting out the external world, so that the wearer may focus on more spiritual concerns.

Business

The blue or grey of the suits worn by many businesspeople – another kind of uniform – convey the impression that these are sober, reliable people whom we can trust with our money or details of our affairs. The colour of the uniforms worn by the staff of many companies is carefully chosen for the qualities associated with it – orange for zest and vitality, red and yellow for energy and stimulation, green for health and so on.

School uniform

Even the colours of the uniforms that some schoolchildren wear – blue, grey, brown, black and so on – are chosen to encourage conformity, rather than to reflect the energies of the individual. Given the constraints imposed upon many of us by the colour we have to wear to work, it is small wonder that the first thing we do when we get home is to change into a colour in which we feel we can be more ourselves.

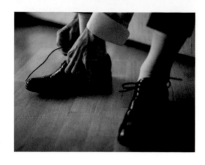

Personal touch
Even if you wear a uniform at work, or clothes that conform to other people's expectations, you can still complement what you wear with an accessory – a tie, ring, scarf or belt – in a colour that you particularly like.

WHAT COLOUR DO YOU WEAR? The fabric of the clothes
that we wear acts as a filter for colour to be absorbed through the skin. For example, if you are wearing a green shirt, then you take in the properties of the colour green. This gives rise to a sense of harmony with your surroundings and opens you up. It is therefore important that the colours you choose to wear reflect or enhance your natural energies, which of course vary from day to day.

What you don't wear
Think about the colour you never wear, that's not represented in your wardrobe, and its particular properties. Refer to Chapter 2 (pages 22–93) if you want to refresh your memory about the colours and what they stand for. If, for example, you never wear red, is it because you are naturally a 'red' person and don't need that energy, or is it because you're lacking in energy, confidence or initiative? If it is the latter, then wearing red can help you to develop these qualities.

Questionnaire

What colour do you always wear?

How do you feel in it?

How do others react to you in it?

What colour do you never wear? Why?

What colour are you wearing now? Why did you choose it?

When you look at all your clothes, what colours dominate?

What colours are missing from your clothing collection?

Look at the clothes that you don't wear any more, what colour are they?

What colour would you like to wear but don't? Why not?

Have you recently bought something in a new colour? What prompted you to do this?

Dark, bright or neutral?

We tend to wear dark colours when we feel physically or emotionally low, bright colours when we are in high spirits and neutral colours when we are tired and want to take it easy. The questionnaire on the left is designed to make you think about the colours that you wear or don't wear, so take a few moments to answer it using paper and pen.

Dark colours

Bright colours

Neutral colours

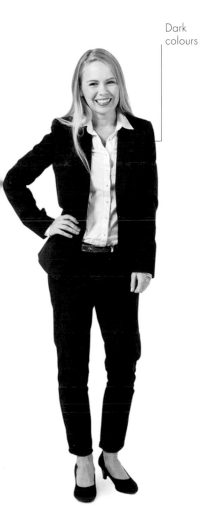
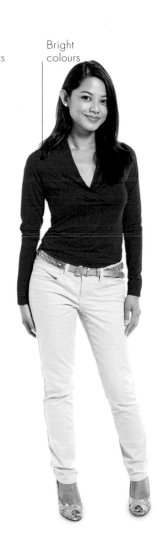
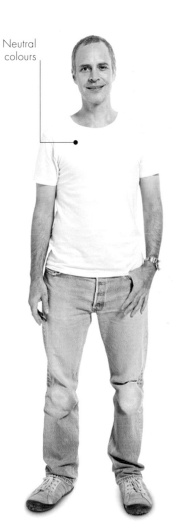

Your Natural Colouring

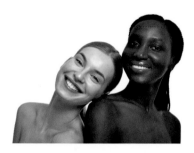

Skin colour
What goes with the colour of your skin influences the colours that you choose to wear.

Most of us, whether consciously or unconsciously, choose colours to wear that go with our natural colouring, i.e. the colour of our skin, eyes and hair. If we wear colours that clash with these, then we tend not to look our best and other people are quite likely to say that those particular colours do not suit us.

A German colour theorist, Johannes Itten, categorized people of different colouring according to the four seasons of the year – spring, summer, autumn and winter. While not everyone falls neatly into these categories because we may be of mixed race or given to experimenting with the colour of our hair – or even our eyes, in the form of coloured contact

lenses – they serve as a useful guide to the colours in which each of us looks and feels good. Read on to discover which season you fit into, and the colours that suit you best.

'Spring' & 'summer' people

'Spring' people tend to have pink/ivory skin – the English 'peaches-and-cream' complexion is typical of this – blue or green eyes and golden blonde or brown hair. They look good in light, pale colours such as pink, peach, lemon, cream and green. These people are often lively, outgoing and enthusiastic.

'Summer' people are also fair-skinned and often have pink complexions, commonly with pale blue or grey, but sometimes hazel, eyes and light blonde or brown hair. The colours that look best on them are blue and pink. Summer people are dependable, cooperative, sensitive and serious.

'Autumn' & 'winter' people

The colouring of 'autumn' people tends to be that of their season – red, brown and gold. Their skin tone usually ranges from golden through tan to copper, and they also often have freckles. Their eyes are usually green or brown and their hair shades of red or brown. People of this type look best in rich autumn colours – orange, yellow and russet.

Many 'winter' people are olive- or dark-skinned and have eyes of varying shades of brown. Their hair is usually dark brown or black. People of this type look good in strong, bright colours such as red, green or purple, but they are also particularly suited to wearing black or white.

Chinese Seasons

In traditional Chinese medicine, each season has an associated colour and element, which is linked to parts of the body. Each seasonal type of person therefore has a tendency to weakness in certain health areas. For winter people, these include the urinary system; for spring people, the liver; for summer people, the heart; for autumn people, the lungs.

COLOURS FOR LEISURE WEAR

While the clothes we wear to the office may have to conform to the colours of the company or the institution that employs us, away from the workplace we can wear the colours that we particularly like. There are colours, however, that are especially good for certain activities. Whatever you decide to do with your leisure time, the colours that you wear can not only help to reflect your mood, but can also help to create it.

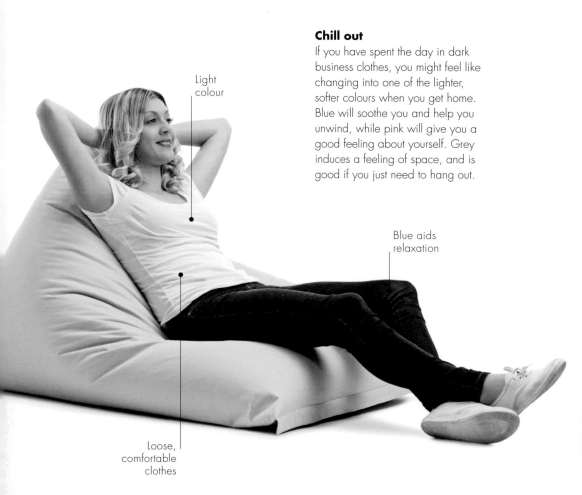

Light colour

Loose, comfortable clothes

Chill out

If you have spent the day in dark business clothes, you might feel like changing into one of the lighter, softer colours when you get home. Blue will soothe you and help you unwind, while pink will give you a good feeling about yourself. Grey induces a feeling of space, and is good if you just need to hang out.

Blue aids relaxation

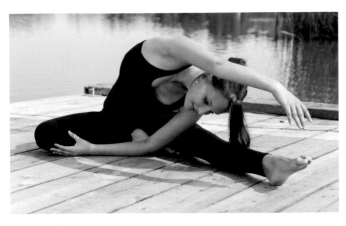

Sociable Colours

The colours at the warm end of the spectrum are also good to wear if you are socializing after work and want to liven yourself up.

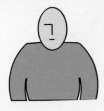

Red or orange

Red will give you the confidence to go up to people that you do not know, and orange will put you in a party mood.

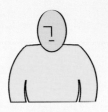

Yellow

Yellow will get you talking to others.

Energy boost

If you are one of those people who likes to go to the gym or for a run after work, you might opt to change into an energetic colour like red or orange, particularly if you have had a tiring day. They will give you the boost that you need for strenuous physical exercise.

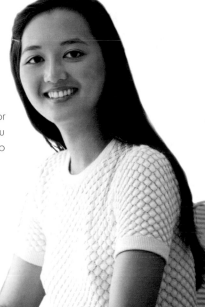

Mental stimulation

If you intend to spend the evening studying, perhaps for a course or an exam that you are taking, you might want to put on something yellow, to stimulate your mind.

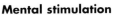

Natural Versus Synthetic Fibres

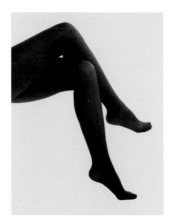

Synthetic material
Many modern clothes are made of synthetic material, but the skin cannot breathe through them.

It is not only the colour that we wear that is important to our well-being, but also the quality of the fabric itself. Whether a fabric is natural or synthetic will make a very big difference to how we feel when wearing it.

Synthetic, or man-made, fibres have been popular since World War II, because they make possible the manufacture of mass-market clothing at prices everyone can afford. Nylon, the first and best known of the synthetic fibres, has become synonymous with one of the products for which it is used, ladies' stockings.

However, synthetic fibres are produced by chemically processing raw materials like wood pulp and petroleum extracts and these do not allow the skin to breathe. Also, light cannot penetrate the fabric in the same way as through natural fibres.

Silk
Perhaps the most sensuous of natural fibres is silk, and after thousands of years of people wearing it, it is still considered a luxury material. Silk is the stuff of cocoons that are made by certain species of caterpillars and for many centuries its main producer, China, shrouded its production in secrecy. Apart from its sheen and softness to the touch, silk has another important quality: its fibres reflect light like a prism and it has high absorbency, enabling it to be dyed with a range of deep, brilliant colours. This makes silk one of the most effective fabric conductors of colour energy.

Cotton
Cotton is one of the most common of all textile fibres and its history goes back thousands of years. A product of the cotton plant, it is a clean, fresh fabric that feels very comfortable next to the skin.

Cotton is very versatile, because it can be woven in any texture and dyed in any colour. It allows the skin to breathe, and light to reach the skin.

Wool

Wool is a fibre that is made from the fleece or hair of various animals and it can include alpaca, mohair, cashmere and camel. The making of wool was a major industry in ancient Babylon and Mesopotamia. Wool contains tiny air pockets that insulate the body and it is also easy to dye. It too, lets in light and so allows the body to absorb colour.

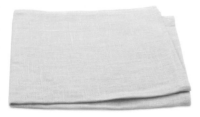

Presentation skills
If you have an important presentation
to make and therefore want to express
yourself clearly in order to get your
message across, try adding a touch
of yellow to what you are wearing.

COLOURS FOR WORKWEAR
The colour that you wear at work
depends to some extent on the conventions of business dress – this has traditionally
been narrower for men than for women, since women can generally get away with
wearing much brighter colours. However, this is now changing and the most important
points to consider are what your career is, and what impression you want to create.

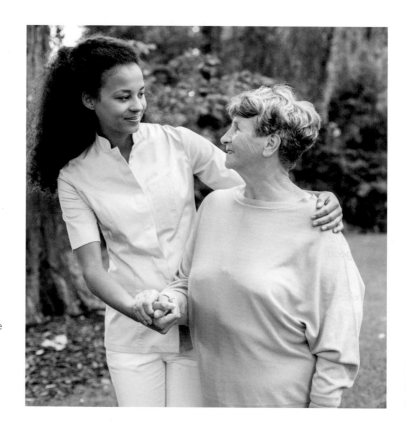

Approachability
If your job involves a lot of
direct dealing with people,
perhaps in a helping or
counselling capacity, it is
best to wear softer, warmer
colours. Pink or peach, for
example, will help people
to feel comfortable with you.
Green, blue and turquoise are
also good colours to wear
because they will help you
to empathize with people
and give you an insight
into their problems.

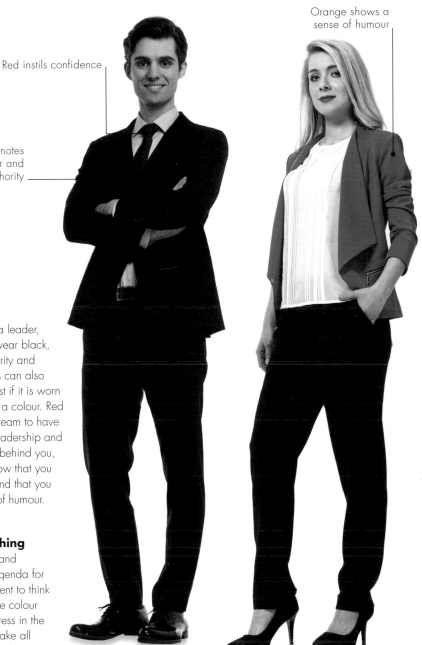

Orange shows a
sense of humour

Red instils confidence

Black denotes
power and
authority

Leadership

If your role is that of a leader,
you may choose to wear black,
which bestows authority and
power. However, this can also
intimidate, so it is best if it is worn
with an accessory in a colour. Red
will encourage your team to have
confidence in your leadership and
will get them pulling behind you,
while orange will show that you
are young at heart and that you
have a good sense of humour.

Appropriate clothing

Whatever your job, and
whatever is on the agenda for
the day, take a moment to think
about the appropriate colour
to wear when you dress in the
morning – it could make all
the difference to your day.

Colours That You Don't Wear

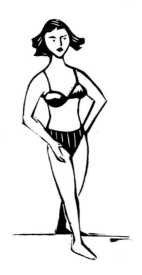

Underwear
*The colour of your underwear
can also help you feel the
way you want to.*

The colour that you don't wear could be the colour to which you need to pay the most attention. It may well be that you have outgrown it now; it represents a stage in your life that you have moved on from and that's why you no longer wear clothes of that colour. If you have a pile of clothes that you have not worn for a year, either because they do not fit well, are no longer fashionable, you do not like them or you no longer like the colour, then get rid of them. Take them to a charity shop or give them to a friend so they don't clutter up your life any more.

Colours that fight back

Alternatively, it may be that you tend to express the negative side of the qualities that the particular colour represents. It could be yellow: when this energy is working well in you, you think clearly, the ideas come and you communicate well with others. But if it's not, you may find yourself continually picking fault with other people and taking a cynical view of things, which makes you unpopular. You may not have the skin tone for yellow – it goes best with sallow or darker-coloured skin – but you can always wear a touch of yellow (for example, a scarf) as an accessory to help you develop the colour's positive traits.

Colour compromises

If you really dislike a colour and cannot see yourself in it at all, you can always wear it as underwear. For example, maybe you feel red is just too much for you to wear, but at the same time you want to become more assertive at work. Try wearing some red underwear to help you stand up for yourself. It will also keep you warm.

You can also wear a shade or a tint of the colour that you don't like – choose pink or magenta as a substitute for red; apricot or peach instead of orange; and lilac or lavender as a replacement for purple. A substitute shade or tint will not have as strong an effect as the unadulterated colour, but it will still influence the way that you feel.

However, it's important that you don't wear a colour that you don't like simply because it happens to be in fashion: follow your heart rather than the dictates of fashion (and that goes for choice of clothes, too).

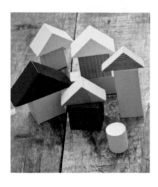

Building blocks
Look around your personal environment with fresh eyes and think about the colour you live with, so that it truly reflects the colour you are.

COLOURS THAT YOU LIVE WITH Our own home is where we take sanctuary from the world; we return to it at the end of a day's work, and also eat, sleep, make love, relax with family and friends and recuperate after illness there. In short, it is the place where we spend a large part of our lives and so it's important that the colour we live with supports us physically, emotionally, mentally and spiritually.

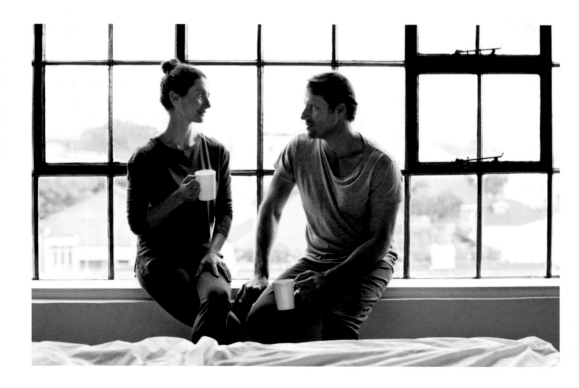

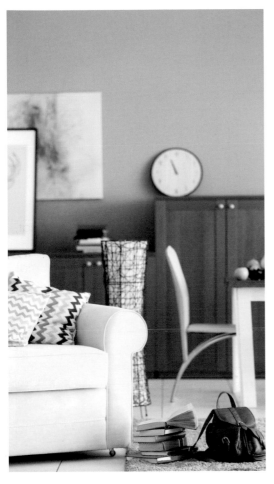

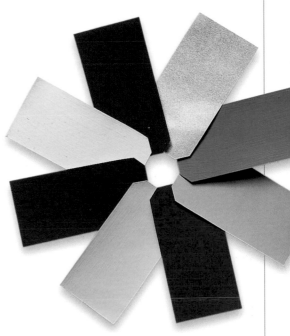

Paint samples
If you want some ideas, walk around your home with a swatch of paint samples.

Colour transformations

You may not have given much thought to the colours you are surrounded by; you may have lived with the same colours for years, never really taking them in or pausing to consider whether they truly reflect who you are. At the same time you may be aware of not liking a particular room, because it's too small, too dark or too cold. Colour can help to transform such an environment, turning a room you avoid, or use for storing junk, into a space that supports you in whatever activity you choose to do in there.

Follow your instincts

You don't have to spend a fortune on materials or interior designers to get your home looking the way you want it to. Paint can be obtained inexpensively and most of us can pick up a brush and slap some on a wall. The important thing is to choose the colours you want, not what is fashionable or what other people think you should have. Your favorite colour, or a colour you need to have around you to reflect who you are at a particular time in your life, may be a colour that someone else can't stand.

What Colours Do You Live With?

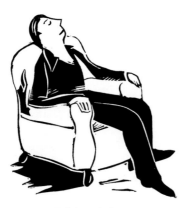

Taking it in
Have a good look round the place where you live and take in all the colours.

Take a few moments with pen and paper to answer the questionnaire on the next page. You could also try wandering through the rooms in your flat or house, looking around you at the colour you live with and thinking about the questions asked. Look up and down as well as around you – look at the ceiling above your head and the floor beneath your feet. You should also take in the furnishings, pictures and books on the shelves and check your instinctive reaction to the colours you see. Is there too much

of one colour? Not enough of another? Is the overall effect too dark, too light, too bright or too dull?

It may be that as you look around you, a colour comes into your mind – remember it; it may be a colour that you need at this point in your life, to reflect a change in yourself or your circumstances. Perhaps, for example, you now work from home instead of going out to an office; or maybe someone has moved in, or out.

What the room is for

You also need to consider what each room is for and whether its colour scheme serves that purpose. Take your bedroom, for example. How well do you sleep in it? Do you wake up refreshed in the morning after a good night's sleep or do you surface feeling tired after waking up in the middle of the night and tossing and turning? If the latter, it may be that your bedroom is in one of the colours at the warm end of the spectrum, which are very stimulating, while you need a cool, calm blue. You can ask yourself the same kind of question for each room as you go around your home. Is the living room a place where people relax and talk or is it somewhere they argue? How much work do you get done in your study? What colour would help to change things? Refer to Chapter 2 (pages 22–93) if you're not sure what particular colour to use, but, above all, be guided by your own intuition.

Questionnaire

What is the main colour of the room you are in?

How do you feel in this room?

How do other members of your family/friends behave in this room? Do they act aggressively? Are they restless or relaxed?

Is it in a colour you like? If not, what colour would you change it to?

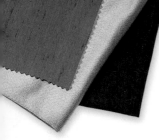

Complementary colours
Colours can be used not only on their own, but also to complement each other.

LIVING ROOM & BEDROOM
The living room is one of the focal areas in any home; it's the place where the occupants congregate, socialize, watch TV, read and generally 'hang out'. So it's a room that has to perform several different functions, all of which need to be taken into account when planning its colour scheme.

Creating an atmosphere

The main thing to consider when you begin to plan is what kind of atmosphere you wish to create – whether you wish it to be quiet and peaceful, or warm and welcoming. If the latter, you will need to introduce colours from the warm end of the spectrum, perhaps peach or apricot – tints of orange, which is a joyful and expansive colour. Either of these would go well with blue, the complementary colour to orange, and this combination would create an environment in which people can relax in each other's company. The effect can be enhanced by cushions, throws and pictures in varying tones of the two colours.

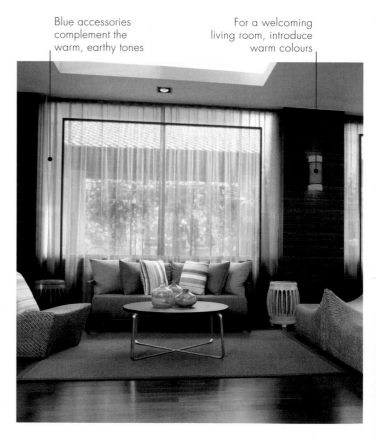

Blue accessories complement the warm, earthy tones

For a welcoming living room, introduce warm colours

A restful room

The bedroom is another very important room because that's where we sleep, make love, think, read and, perhaps, write. It's essentially a private room, whether you retire there to be alone or to be intimate with another person. So it's a room which, perhaps more than any other, needs to be decorated in colours that reflect who you are.

Primarily the colours you use need to be restful so that you can get a good night's sleep. Pink is a popular colour for bedrooms as it's soft and gentle and will make you feel supported. You can also use tints of white rather than white on its own which can look and feel a bit clinical (see pages 80–81). Blue is a tranquil colour, but is not the best choice if your room is cold, because it will make it seem even colder.

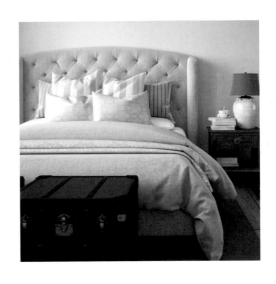

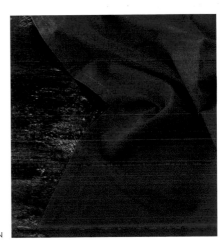

SCENTED CANDLES   OIL BURNER

Passionate touches

If you want to create a setting for passionate lovemaking, you can always introduce red into the decor, although this is best done in the form of sheets or candles and coloured lightbulbs, otherwise you are unlikely to be able to get a good night's sleep.

CANDLE   RED LINEN

Connecting Spaces

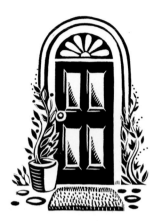

Impression
*Even the colour of your front door will give
your visitors a particular impression.*

There are many other spaces in a house besides rooms and these mainly consist of connecting spaces like entrance halls, staircases, landings and passages. These spaces connect in more than one sense since they are spaces that people move through on their way from one part of the house to another, as well as using them to linger in for a quick chat, a gossip or a hastily imparted confidence.

These spaces are places of activity and are also often the first part of your home that people will see. So, what impression do you want them to get? Dramatic, warm and welcoming, or a haven from the world? Bright, vibrant colours from the warm end of the spectrum will welcome them into your home and make them feel a part of it. If you want to create a softer, cosier effect, you can always use tints or shades of these colours, such as terracotta or rust for red or orange, and lemon for yellow. It is also important to pay attention to the colour that you paint the front door. In some cultures, it is always painted in a protective colour, such as black, white, purple or blue.

If, on the other hand, you work long hours in a demanding job, you may just want to shut the door on the world and collapse when you get home at night. If so, colours from the cool end of the spectrum will help you to unwind the moment you step inside.

Neutral colours

Communal areas are often painted in neutral colours such as off-white, cream or beige, but these can make for a static atmosphere, where strangers visiting your home just huddle inside the front door, not knowing whether to advance or not.

Sometimes these connecting areas of our homes are small, cramped spaces without much natural light and they may also be stuffy and cold. Different colours can help to counter this: pastel colours, for example, will create a light, spacious effect, while dark or rich colours will make a space more intimate. A cold corridor can be made to seem warmer by the use of a colour from the red end of the spectrum. An airless landing will seem cooler and fresher if a colour from the blue end of the spectrum is used.

Feng Shui

According to the Chinese practice of Feng Shui, the position of your staircase affects the chi (energy) present in the house. It is not good if a staircase starts directly in front of the front door. Curving stairs are preferable to straight, spiral staircases are not recommended, and steps should be solid and always covered.

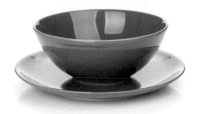

Bright colours
Bright colours in the kitchen will help create a warm, inviting atmosphere.

THE KITCHEN & BATHROOM
The kitchen and bathroom are two contrasting rooms, in which very different kinds of activities take place. The kitchen is not only the place where food is cooked, it is often also where the family gathers together for a meal and where we entertain friends. The bathroom is a much more private room to which we may like to retreat for a long hot soak at the end of a tiring day.

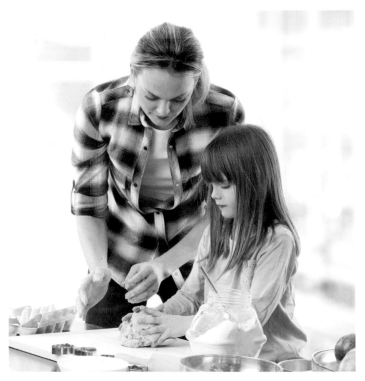

Heart of the home
The kitchen is the hub of the house and so the colours used here need to reflect warmth and conviviality. Red will energize; orange will whet the appetite and aid the digestion; and yellow will stimulate conversation. Red also earths us and so a kitchen floor made up of terracotta tiles, for example, will help us to find our feet after a day spent in front of a computer or at meetings with other people. The kitchen also offers plenty of scope for splashes of contrasting or complementary colour in the form of bowls of fruit and vegetables, plants, displays of crockery and so on.

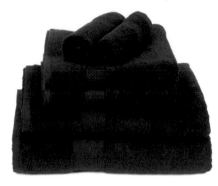

Inviting bathrooms

Many bathrooms are small, poky places without even a window. This makes it even more important to choose colours that will make the room look lighter and larger, such as blues and turquoise, the colours of the sea, which will help to relax and soothe you. The bathroom is not a place where you want to feel cold, however, so these need to be offset by softer, warmer colours in the form of a rug, bathmat, towels or bathrobe.

Blue

Shades of blue in the bathroom will help put you in a relaxing frame of mind.

Warm-toned lamp

Blue and turquoise decor

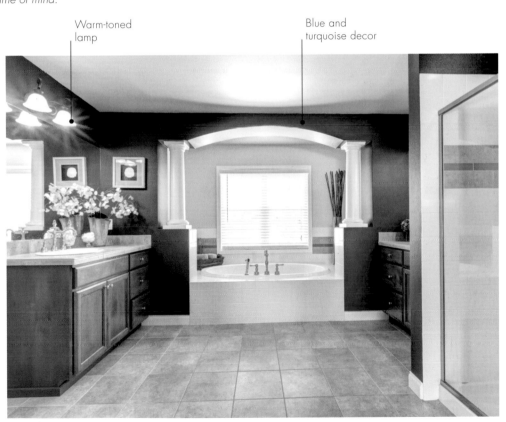

Other Rooms

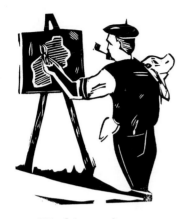

Working at home
The colour of your study or studio can make all the difference to how your work goes.

There are, of course, other rooms in the house, such as a conservatory or study. The study area may be a corner of another room or a loft specially converted for the purpose. Studies are often used for hobbies, or for children to do their homework. Until recently, it was probably considered something of a luxury to have a room in the house devoted entirely to the pursuit of some fascinating hobby. Nowadays, however, as more and more people work from home, it is increasingly a necessity.

Working from home

It may be that you don't have a big enough apartment or house to be able to set aside a room solely for work, but even if you use a space within another room, you still need to think about what colour is going to inspire you and maximize your productivity.

If, for example, your work is of a mental rather than physical nature, involving thinking, reading, writing and coming up with ideas, then yellow is a wonderful colour for stimulating the mind. Being the colour closest to the light of the sun, it will also help to keep up your spirits as you work.

If your work is of an artistic nature – drawing, designing, painting or sewing, for example – then you might want to place purple around you. This is the colour of creative inspiration and it will also help keep the distractions of the outer world at bay.

If space allows, you might want to set aside a corner to rest or meditate, and for this cool blues, greens and turquoise would be best.

Children's rooms

Children very often need an area of their room set aside for study, particularly as they get older. As they grow and develop, they tend to be attracted to stronger and brighter colours, which reflect their abundance of energy. However, these bold, bright colours are not conducive to quiet study, so it is best to partition off a corner of their room and decorate it in paler, softer colours that will encourage them to concentrate when homework has to be done.

If your child experiences difficulty in sleeping, make sure that this is not because the room's colour scheme is too bright and overstimulating.

Pattern Power

Be careful when buying bedding for a child's room. Its colour vibrations will penetrate the aura of a sleeping child. Pay attention to what is printed on the bedding, too. Large, vibrantly coloured designs or bold figures can emit negative vibrational energies.

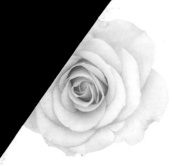

Harmonize with nature

You can create a garden, however small, with colours in it that will change throughout the year to reflect the seasons and your own shifting moods.

COLOUR IN THE GARDEN
Gardens are very healing places, not only because they bring us into contact with nature, but also because of the colours of the plants, flowers and shrubs. Even if you live in the city and can boast only a tiny border and a strip of concrete for a garden, you can still plant it up with colours that will heal and inspire you all year round.

Seasonal colours

Colour does not easily divide into the four seasons of the year any more than many plants do. Yet it is possible to distinguish the pale, promising colours of spring from the brilliant, ripe colours of summer and the dying shades of autumn from the stark contrasts of winter.

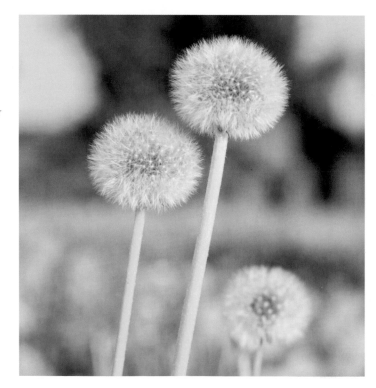

Seasons

Changes in the garden will keep you in touch with the seasons.

Contrasting colours

Complementary colours can work just as well in the garden as in the home.

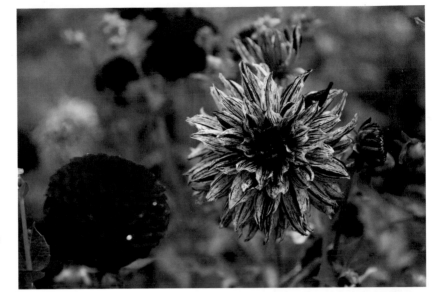

Warm colours

Warm colours like orange can be a joy to look at on a grey day.

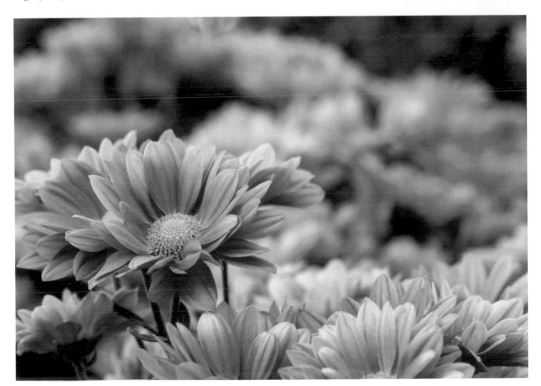

Plants & Flowers for Spring

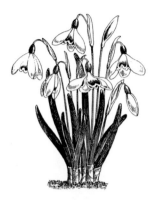

Welcome sight
After the barrenness of winter, the early flowers of spring are a welcome sight.

The flower that we probably associate most with spring is the common snowdrop, whose flowers show dramatically white against the dark ground and bare trees of late winter. But snowdrops can actually flower for up to five months, from autumn and winter to early spring. However, after the long, dark days of winter, they are seen as a herald of the light to come and so we think of them as spring flowers. The shrub magnolia also symbolizes spring, whether it is the pink-flowering variety or *M. stellata*, the star magnolia, so-called because of its star-shaped white flowers. These can be grown in the smallest of gardens and look good planted next to camellias, particularly of the 'Donation' variety. The attractive green foliage and large soft pink flowers of camellias are one of the finest displays of spring.

Azaleas

Azaleas, a form of rhododendron, also flower in late spring and can be grown in large tubs. They come in two varieties, evergreen (also known as Japanese) and deciduous. The colour of the former ranges through most of the colours of the rainbow – from white through pink, red and vermilion to blue, lilac and purple. The deciduous azaleas have a similar range of colours, with the addition of yellow and orange. The species *Rhododendron luteum* produces a golden flower with a particularly fragrant scent.

Spring bulbs

Spring would not be spring without daffodils, narcissi, crocuses and tulips. If you have a large enough garden, create a wild, woodland effect by scattering the bulbs haphazardly under the trees. In spring you will be rewarded by an unforgettable sight.

Crocuses come in many different varieties, in colours ranging from white to golden yellow and purple. Early-flowering tulips come in a similar range of colours, including white and yellow, which are, more than any other, the colours of spring. Some varieties of cyclamen also flower in spring. They vary from white to pink and deep red.

Daffodils

Daffodils are adaptable plants that are happy in shady areas as well as in full sun. Plant the bulbs to a depth of twice the height of the bulb, spacing them 10–20 centimetres (4–8in) apart, in early to mid-autumn. They are best planted in groups or drifts. Let the leaves die back naturally after flowering.

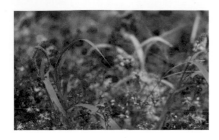

Ablaze with colour
Summer is a time when the garden is ablaze with colour from many different plants.

THE GARDEN IN SUMMER
Summer is a long season, spanning late spring and early autumn. This is reflected in the colours of summer, which range from the pastels of spring to the rich warm colours of autumn. At the height of this season, colour in the garden really comes into its own, as there is an overwhelming variety of herbaceous plants of all kinds and colours as well as a myriad of greens from trees in full leaf.

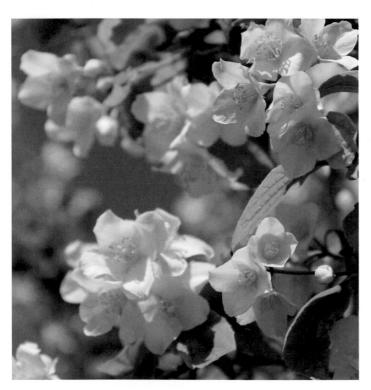

Blossoming forth

In late spring the first roses can already be seen and many shrubs are also coming into season. Geraniums, are starting to bud and a host of annuals are producing their first flowers. In early summer, the day is at its longest and lightest and the garden is bursting with growth of every kind. Midsummer brings forth the climbers – rose, clematis and jasmine – in a tangle of white, pink and blue, while in late summer the later-flowering plants are beginning to take over the garden. By early autumn it's time to plant ahead.

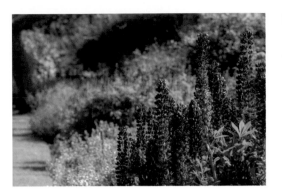

Herbaceous plants

Herbaceous plants, perennials which flower for several years at least, come into their own during the summer months.

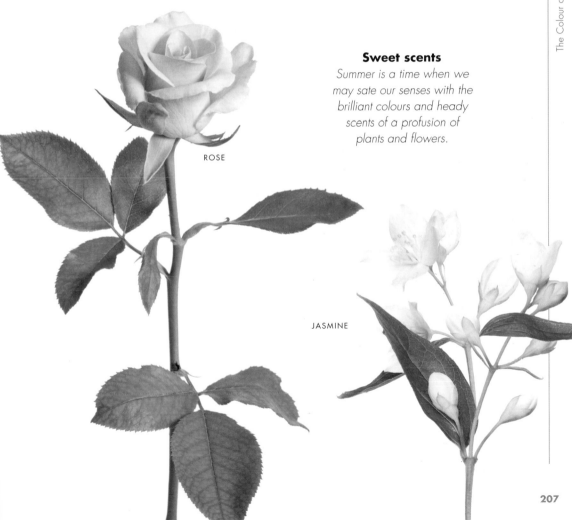

Sweet scents

Summer is a time when we may sate our senses with the brilliant colours and heady scents of a profusion of plants and flowers.

ROSE

JASMINE

Plants & Flowers for Summer

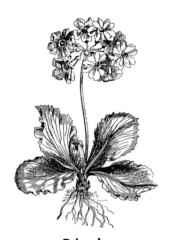

Primula
The primula will grow in most gardens and helps to postpone the end of summer.

Reigning supreme over summer is the rose, which ranges in colour from deep red to yellow and creamy white. The flowers may be single or what are known as full doubles, where the petals are packed together in layers to form a soft, cushiony, sensuous ball. Many varieties also have a divine scent, which is enough to send the senses reeling. Roses are generally at their best in early to midsummer, although some varieties have a second, less fulsome flowering later in the year.

A subtler fragrance is emitted by the small, delicate, pale mauve-pink flowers of the jasmine 'Stephanense', which is often to be found growing side by side with the common white jasmine, which flowers all summer long. Another popular climber is the clematis, which comes in a variety of colours from white, light and dark pink, to blue, mauve and deep purple.

Primulas flower throughout the length of the summer in strong reds, deep purple, yellow and orange. If you have water in your garden, they will do well growing at the edge, since they thrive in a combination of moisture and shade.

Herbaceous plants

Herbaceous plants (those that die back each winter and grow again in spring) provide an endless source of colour throughout the summer months. They include lupins, whose tall spires flower in a range of colours – white, blue, pink, violet, red and yellow – as well as day lilies and carnations. Pink and red sweet williams lend a homely air to the garden, while the vivid red, orange and yellow of California and Iceland poppies light it up.

Hydrangeas

Hydrangeas take us from summer into autumn and reflect the changing of the seasons in their flowers and colours. The flowers' texture goes from silky to waxy and their colours turn from blue to a light pale green, red to brown and from white to greenish-white. There are two kinds of hydrangeas, mopheads – so-called because of their large floppy heads of flowers – and lacecaps, whose flowers are flatter. The mopheads suitable for a small garden are the sky-blue 'Vibraye' and the dwarf 'Pia', whose red flowers take us well into autumn.

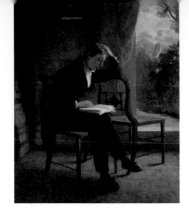

Keats
*The poet wrote of
autumn as 'the season
of mists and mellow
fruitfulness'.*

THE GARDEN IN AUTUMN When there begins to be a chill in
the air and the leaves of the trees start to turn, we know that fall is on its way. The
poignancy of this time of year is heightened by the flare of colour in the foliage of
the trees, which is a final show put on by nature before the light sinks to its lowest
and winter sets in.

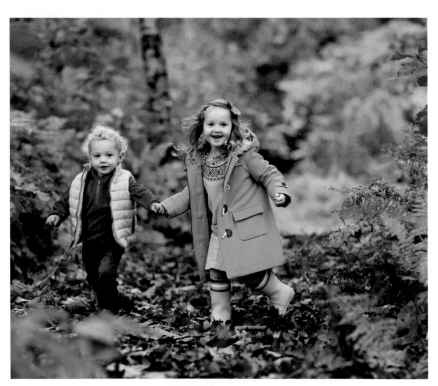

**Autumn
colours**
To take a walk
through woods in
autumn is to be
treated to a blaze
of red, orange,
yellow, gold,
copper and russet,
accentuated by the
green of conifer,
fern and moss.
A shaft of sunlight
striking through the
trees and illumining
the veins of leaves
is a sight to fill us
with awe.

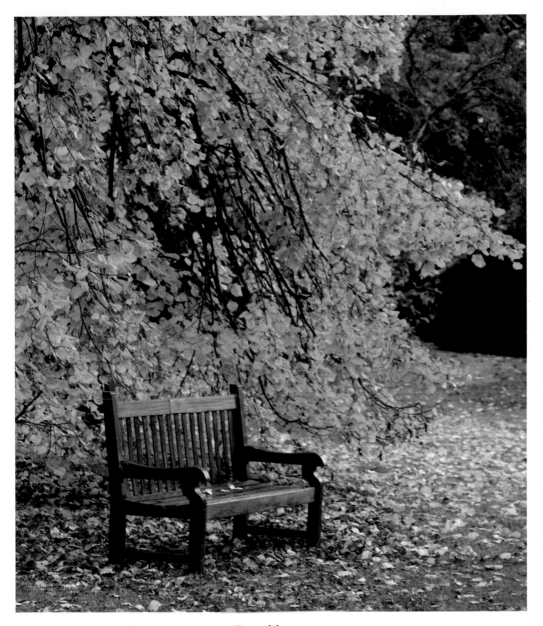

Transition

*Autumn is a time of transition, from ripe
summer to bare winter, when we pause to reflect
on what has passed and what is to come.*

Plants & Flowers for Autumn

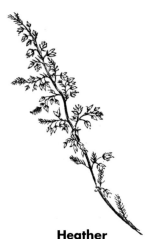

Heather
Heathers flower throughout autumn in colours to match the foliage of the trees.

Some shrubs flower well into fall and among them is the hardy fuchsia, which bears clusters of dangling flowers in a voluptuous magenta. These flowers contrast particularly well with the tall, creamy spikes of the exotic yucca. The hardy hibiscus produces flowers in purplish-red, bluish-purple and white, while an unseasonal and spectacular splash of bright yellow is provided by the evergreen *Hypericum* 'Hidcote'.

Heather is a feature of autumn, and this looks its best when planted massed together, so that the traditional greens and greys we associate with this shrub set off the pink flowers and orange foliage of varieties like 'Orange Queen' or the white flowers and yellow foliage of 'Gold Haze'.

Japanese maples

One of the stars of autumn is undoubtedly the Japanese maple, as its turning leaves provide an unmatched display of rich gold, bright scarlet and canary yellow. The tupelo tree from North America adds orange to this show, while among the mountain ashes the *Sorbus* 'Embley' is renowned for its striking red leaves. The tiny *Sorbus reducta*, which seldom grows to a height of more than 30 centimetres (1 foot), will provide even the smallest of gardens with red and purple autumn colour, as well as white fruits. This is, after all, the season of hips and berries and among the best of the fruiting roses is the *rugosa*, which produces bright red hips the size of small tomatoes.

Autumn bulbs

Autumn-flowering bulbs are not as well known as spring bulbs, with the exception of cyclamen, which flowers pink and white in early autumn. One of the most beautiful bulbs is the nerine, in particular *Nerine bowdenii*, which is hardy and easy to grow. It produces clusters of the most delicate fairy-pink flowers that turn outward at the tips in a feminine curve.

Among autumn-flowering herbaceous plants are Japanese anemones, which range in colour from white and cream to pink and rose. Michaelmas daisies are popular, the most noticeable is *Aster* 'Frikartii', which is distinguished by flowers of a lavender-blue. Finally chrysanthemums create a mass of colour in apricot and bronze, and white, yellow, pink and red.

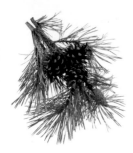

Berries & cones
There may be fewer flowers in winter, but there are berries and cones galore.

THE GARDEN IN WINTER In winter everything seems to come to a standstill. The ground turns hard and may be covered with the white rime of frost or snow, the herbaceous plants have long died, and the deciduous trees and shrubs shed their leaves. Animals hibernate and the days grow shorter and darker.

Winter colour

At this time of year there is little colour from flowers in the garden, but a variety of greens is provided by the conifers and splashes of bright red and yellow by the berries of various shrubs. The black skeletal outlines of trees also contrast sharply with the leaden skies of winter and fallen snow.

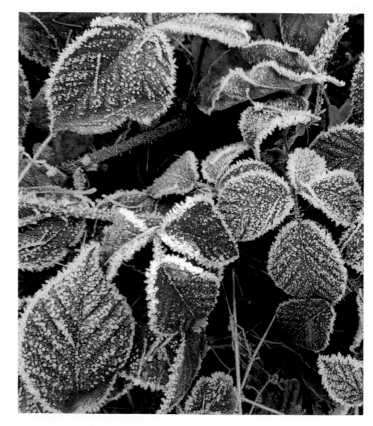

Frost
Winter has its own special beauty, as in these leaves outlined by frost.

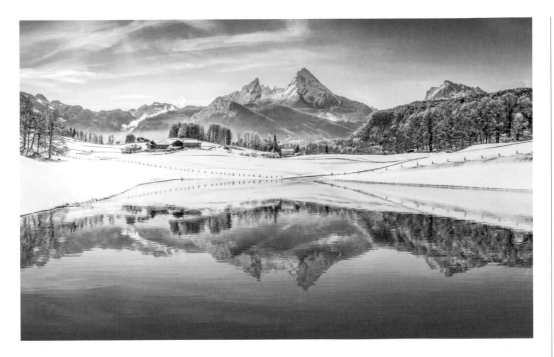

Winter landscape

The whiteness of the snow and the darkness of the Earth throw everything in the winter landscape into sharp definition.

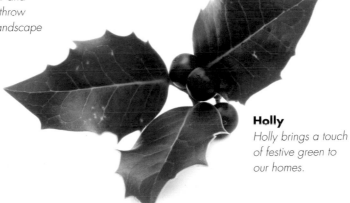

Holly

Holly brings a touch of festive green to our homes.

Conserving energy

Winter is a time for turning inward, whether seated before the leaping flames of a log fire, or on a brisk walk through a mute, starkly beautiful landscape. It is a time for conserving our strength, like the animal and plant life around us, until the light returns in the spring.

Plants & Flowers for Winter

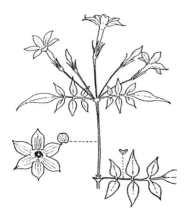

Standing out
Colour in winter stands out all the more for being scarcer than at other times.

The cold, crisp air of winter is scented by the large white or cream flowers of the hybrid honeysuckle as well as by daphnes, whose purplish-pink flowers are followed by black fruits, and the viburnum 'Dawn', whose red buds open to white flowers flushed with pink. Lighting the darkness of winter with its large yellow flowers is the winter jasmine, which looks its best when trailed over a trellis or wall. The evergreen clematis also flowers all winter long, producing blooms of a whitish-yellow. Winter colour is also provided by crocuses in white, pale and dark yellow, blue, mauve and purple as well as by winter-flowering pansies, which range from white to a rich, dark red.

Mahonias are particularly noticeable for their striking evergreen foliage. One of the most beautiful is *Mahonia japonica*, whose stiff, spiny leaves are complemented by clusters of pendulous yellow flowers. This mahonia will flower throughout winter and also bears berries of purple or black.

Holly & ivy

If there is a dearth of colour from flowers in winter, it is in part made up for by the berries that are produced by various shrubs. Pyracanthas, which will grow in almost any soil, produce a wealth of red, orange and yellow fruits throughout the winter. Other berrying shrubs include cotoneaster and of course holly, which is synonymous with the great festival of winter, Christmas. There are many species of holly with a variety of leaves, ranging from the large, shiny and spineless evergreen to the variegated gold kind. We tend to think of the berries as red, but they can also be yellow.

Ivies come into their own during the winter and their leaves trail everywhere in a range of variegated colours – green, yellow, silver, grey and white. They go well with holly, as celebrated in the carol 'The Holly and the Ivy', and a traditional Christmas would seem incomplete without these two stalwarts of winter.

Hellebores

An ideal variety of hellebore for a winter planting is *Helleborus niger*, the Christmas rose. It thrives in shady areas, lighting them up with large white flowers with golden stamens, which bloom from midwinter to early spring.

FURTHER READING

Anderson, Mary, *Colour Healing*, The Aquarian Press, 1990.

Bailey, Nick, *365 Days of Colour in Your Garden*, Kyle Books, 2015.

Cayce, Edgar, *Auras, An Essay on the Meaning of Colours*, A.R.E Press, 1999.

Chiazzari, Suzy, *The Complete Book of Colour*, Element, 1998.

Dalichow, Irene and Booth, Mike, *Aura-Soma, Healing Through Colour, Plant and Crystal Energy*, Hay House Inc., 2004.

Gimbel, Theo, *Healing With Colour*, Gaia Books Ltd., 1997.

Gimbel, Theo, *The Colour Therapy Workbook*, Element, 2002.

Hall, Judy, *The Crystal Bible Volume 1*, Godsfield Press, 2009.

Hall, Judy, *TThe Little Book of Crystals*, Gaia Books Ltd., 2016.

Lacy, Marie Louise, *Know Yourself Through Colour*, The Aquarian Press, 1989.

Lacy, Marie Louise, *The Power of Colour to Heal the Environment*, Rainbow Bridge Publications, 1996.

Ouseley, S.G.J., *Colour Meditations*, Pilgrims Publishing, 2002.

Sun, Howard & Dorothy, *Colour Your Life*, Piatkus, 2013.

Verner-Bonds, Lilian, *New Colour Healing*, Vermilion, 2002.

Wall, Vicky, *Aura-Soma: Self-Discovery through Color*, Healing Arts Press, 2005.

USEFUL ADDRESSES

Aura-Soma Products Ltd.
South Road Tetford Horncastle
Lincs. LN9 6QB UK.
Tel: 01507 533581.
Fax: 01507 533412.
info@aura-soma.net
www.aura-soma.net

Aura-Soma USA
North America Aura-Soma LLC
1027 Longdraw Dr.
Katy TX 77494
U.S.A.
Tel: 832-647-5687
debbie@northamerica-
aurasoma.com
www.northamerica-aurasoma.
com/

Aura-Soma Australia
PO Box 4025
Illawong
NSW 2234
Tel: (02) 9541 1066
www.aura-soma.com.au

**International Association
of Colour**
77 Holders Hill Drive
Hendon, London NW4 1NN
England, UK
Tel: 0208 3493299
lilianvernerbonds@yahoo.com
www.iac-colour.co.uk

**The Complementary
Medical Association**
www.the-cma.org.uk

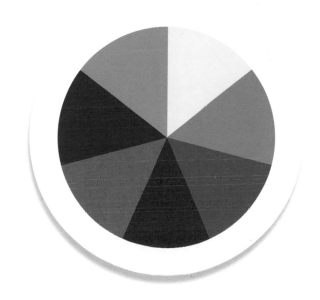

INDEX

ACKNOWLEDGEMENTS

I wish to thank Dolores for all she has taught me over the years; my sister Felicité, and Zena for their help; and Anne, for her delicious recipes and especially for her support and encouragement.

The publisher would like to thank Helene Enahoro, Ian Louis-Fernand, Helen Furbear, Elizabeth Gough, Tara Grant, Emma Hockridge, J. Kinchett, Ben Lacey, Karen Legg, Kay Macmullan, Janina Sanders, Lorraine Torres, for help with photography.

PICTURE ACKNOWLEDGEMENTS

Every effort has been made to trace copyright holders and obtain permission.
The publishers apologize for any omissions and would be pleased to make any necessary changes at subsequent printings

Alamy/ Chronicle: 13; Ian Dagnall: 14B; Cairney Down: 70B; Emotive Images: 125; GL Archive: 16; Granger Historical Picture Archive: 123T; Heritage Image Partnership Ltd: 58B; INTERFOTO: 117; Pictorial Press Ltd: 84; Simon Reddy: 172; Westend61 GmbH: 156. **Bridgeman Images**/ Private Collection / Photo © Christie's Images: 34T. **Getty**/ Martin Barraud: 144; DU CANE MEDICAL IMAGING LTD/SCIENCE PHOTO LIBRARY: 46B; GARION HUTCHINGS/SCIENCE PHOTO LIBRARY: 97; Kean Collection / Staff: 8; Chris Walsh: 31BL; Wavebreakmedia Ltd: 127B. **iStock**/ 4x6: 83B, 143; aldomurillo: 27BR; KatarzynaBialasiewicz: 201; bluejayphoto: 215T; bravo1954: 142T; drbimages: 59B, 63B; francescoch: 101; Gokcemim: 198T; Gromovataya: 78T; GSPictures: 21; Hixson: 42; KariHoglund : 98T; ilbusca: 77; jaboo2foto: 109; kupicoo : 190B; NeilLang: 211; Ljupco : 182; londoneye: 43B, 103; malerapaso: 175; Maxiphoto: 98B; Josef Mohyla: 183T; Neyya: 89; NoDerog: 82T; OSTILL: 27TL; PIKSEL: 51B; powerofforever: 11; Rawpixel: 179; Renphoto: 37; Rike_: 157; sdominick: 2; ShutterWorx: 194B; starush: 83T; Szepy: 199B; VladimirFLoyd: 19B. **Library of Congress**/ 66B. **Shutterstock**/ 2M media: 195T; Africa Studio: 191L, 193; Aila Images: 79B; Ayman Alakhras: 199T; Potapov Alexander: 207BR; AlinaMD: 161; Stefania Arca: 119TL; arindambanerjee: 9; artpritsadee: 158T; BABAROGA: 102B; BasPhoto: 18T; Angyalosi Beata: 195BC; Anna Bogush: 195BR; Artazum: 199B; bigacis: 162L; bikeriderlondon: 29, 121; Bildagentur Zoonar GmbH: 86–87, 185, 217; Bình Thanh Bùi: 38T; bitt24: 159T; Boule: 173; natalia bulatova: 190T; Supavadee butradee: 209; Capricorn Studio: 54B; Capture Light: 15B; Chireau: 25; CHOATphotographer: 114T; Alex Coan: 171TR; ColoArt: 122T; Paolo Costa: 70T; Elizabeth A.Cummings: 170C; Da-ga: 167BR; DaLiu: 165; Daxiao Productions: 75B; Aekkaphop Deehlai: 147T; Del Boy: 50BL; Didecs: 39T, 43T, 47T, 51T, 55T, 59T, 63T, 67T, 71T; Digiart CT: 68; Dionisvera: 162R; DLameko: 62T; Dundanim: 26L; DW labs Incorporated: 154; East: 118T; Tiffany Egbert: 203T; ESB Professional: 167T; FamVeld: 210B; Kostiantyn Fastov: 171B; SvetlanaFedoseyeva: 180; Igor Filonenko: 31; fizkes: 135, 136, 139; Blaj Gabriel: 47B; gudak: 38B; Hesvald: 58T; hjochen: 133; JIANG HONGYAN: 45, 171C; ideafactory250: 181; Tarasyuk Igor: 163C; ImageFlow: 90T; Ivaylo Ivanov: 166T; Izmael: 82B; jiangdi: 170T; joesayhello: 158B; jorisvo: 62B; josehidalgo87: 142B; Julian52000: 213; Vipada Kanajod: 194T; Evgeny Karandaev: 198T; kai keisuke: 19CL; Nikola Knezevic: 110BR; Alexey Kotikov: 41; Lapina: 187R; Johan Larson: 26R; Henrik Larsson: 147B; lenetstan: 155B; LifetimeStock: 34B; Martin Lisner: 169; Lithiumphoto: 159B; Nadya Lukic: 79T; Maodice: 134B; MaraZe: 168; Mike Mareen: 91T; Quinn Martin: 206T; Benny Marty : 177; Lorant Matyas: 74B; Lena May: 65; mbolina: 108; MestoSveta: 184; Anatolii Mikhailov: 202B; MimaCZ: 135; Monkey Business Images: 183B; Morphart Creation: 129; Moving Moment: 167BR; mubus7: 167BL; Niyom Napalai: 149; Maks Narodenko: 50T, 162T; Antonio Nardelli: 163TL; NASA images: 30TR, 31, 31TR; Dmitry Naumov: 50BR; Neirfy: 205; Nejron Photo: 57; Nicolesa: 197; Mr.Cheangchai Noojuntuk: 102T; Nostalgia for Infinity: 31BR; Titima Ongkantong: 96; Kateryna Ovcharenko: 146B; Paperboat: 91B; pathdoc: 76; Evgenii Pavlov: 6T; Pefkos: 215B; Dasha Petrenko: 81; Photick: 61; PhotoEd: 166BR; photofriend: 214T; Photographee.eu: 186B; PhotoMediaGroup: 105; pinkomelet: 189; Pixus: 30; Ploipiroon: 202T; Pogarytskyy: 100; Polygraphus: 49; postolit: 195C; Pressmaster: 138B; racorn: 53; rangizzz: 30FL; ravipat: 93; rprongjai: 166BL; Benjavisa Ruangvaree: 134T; Manfred Ruckszio: 214B; George Rudy: 141; Oleksandr Rybitskiy: 155T; Vadim Sadovski: 30; sakdam: 120; Roman Samborskyi: 99; samodelkin8: 66T; Sarah2: 42T; shooarts: 145; PavelShynkarou: 80; Tanya Sid: 186T; siloto: 113; Viorel Sima: 55B, 187L; s_maria: 167T; Soyka: 207BL; studiovin: 110T; Susii: 54T; Svetlana Serebryakova: 163B; Joy Tasa: 203B; Tethys Imaging LLC: 69; thatmacroguy: 207T; Tiger Images: 170B; timquo: 195BL; TinasDreamworld: 164; Travel_ Master: 73; Tridsanu Thopet: 23; Tristan3D: 30B; Undrey: 27BL; uzhursky: 178T; colin robert varndell: 147C; Gorbash Varvara: 95; Yuliyan Velchev: 46T; yana_vinnikova: 163BL; VladKK: 137; Vvoe: 86T; Krailurk Warasup: 42B; Wire_man: 14T; HWisch: 78B; yoshi0511: 33; Davydenko Yuliia: 163TR; IhorZigor: 74T; Sergey Zlobin: 206B.